The Carnivore Diet

Complete Guide

Polly Olson

Content

Charter 1. Introduction

What is the Carnivore Diet?

The carnivore diet, in its essence, is the practice of consuming exclusively animal-based foods while completely eliminating all plant-based foods from one's diet. This means that followers eat only meat, fish, eggs, and certain dairy products, depending on the variation they choose to follow. The diet has gained popularity in recent years, but its roots and philosophy trace back much further.

A Brief History of the Carnivore Diet

While the carnivore diet might seem like a modern fad to some, its origins are deeply embedded in human history. Early humans, particularly those living in colder climates during the Paleolithic era, relied heavily on animal foods for survival. With limited access to plant foods during harsh winters, hunting and consuming large game became essential. Indigenous populations like the Inuit and Maasai have traditionally consumed diets predominantly composed of animal products, thriving on them for generations.

In the 19th century, Arctic explorer Vilhjalmur Stefansson lived among the Inuit and adopted their all-meat diet, later reporting excellent health and vitality. His experiences challenged the conventional wisdom of the time, which emphasized the importance of fruits and vegetables for preventing diseases like scurvy. Stefansson's accounts sparked interest and scientific studies into the viability of an all-meat diet for human health.

Defining the Carnivore Diet

The carnivore diet is more than just a meal plan; it's a radical departure from the standard dietary guidelines that emphasize a balance of macronutrients from both plant and animal sources. By focusing solely on animal products, the diet eliminates all carbohydrates, relying entirely on proteins and fats for energy. This approach is grounded in the belief that human physiology is better adapted to meat consumption and that many modern ailments stem from plant-based foods.

There are several variations of the carnivore diet, each differing in strictness:

1. Strict Carnivore Diet: This form involves consuming only red meat—primarily beef—and water. Advocates believe that red meat provides all the necessary nutrients and that simplifying the diet aids in digestion and reduces inflammation.

2. Moderate Carnivore Diet: This variation includes a broader range of animal foods such as pork, poultry, fish, and eggs. It allows for more variety while still excluding all plant-based foods.

3. Carnivore Diet with Dairy: Adding dairy products like cheese, butter, and ghee introduces additional fats and flavors. Some followers include dairy to increase their intake of certain nutrients like calcium and vitamin D.

4. Carnivore-ish Diet: This flexible approach primarily focuses on animal foods but permits small amounts of non-animal products. It may include spices, herbs, and even occasional low-carb plant foods to enhance meal enjoyment and sustainability.

Comparison with Other Diets

The carnivore diet shares some similarities with other low-carb, high-fat diets but differs in significant ways:

- **Ketogenic Diet:** Both diets aim to shift the body's metabolism from relying on carbohydrates to burning fats for fuel, leading to a state of ketosis. However, the ketogenic diet allows for low-carb vegetables, nuts, and seeds, whereas the carnivore diet eliminates all plant foods.

- **Paleo Diet:** The paleo diet focuses on eating whole foods that our Paleolithic ancestors might have consumed, including meat, fish, fruits, vegetables, nuts, and seeds. It excludes processed foods, grains, and legumes but is more plant-inclusive than the carnivore diet.
- **Atkins Diet:** Similar to the ketogenic diet, the Atkins diet is low in carbohydrates but permits a gradual increase in carb intake over time. It includes a variety of food groups, unlike the carnivore diet's exclusive focus on animal products.

Philosophy Behind Consuming Only Animal Products

Proponents of the carnivore diet argue that many health issues arise from consuming plant toxins, anti-nutrients, and excessive carbohydrates found in plant foods. They believe that an all-meat diet can reduce inflammation, improve digestion, and lead to better overall health. The diet is often touted for its simplicity—by eating only animal products, individuals can more easily control their nutrient intake and avoid processed foods.

Additionally, some followers report mental health benefits, such as improved mood and cognitive function, attributing these changes to stable blood sugar levels and the absence of inflammatory plant compounds.

Carnivore Diet as a Good Start

A carnivore diet can be an excellent starting point for those interested in radically transforming their eating habits. By focusing on nutrient-dense, satiating foods, individuals may find it easier to adhere to the diet and experience weight loss, improved energy levels, and other health benefits.

For those hesitant to dive into a strict carnivore regimen, beginning with a carnivore-ish approach allows for a gradual transition. Incorporating elements like gravies, sugar-free snacks, or minimal plant-based garnishes can make the diet more palatable and sustainable in the long term. This flexibility can help ease the body into metabolic changes and reduce potential side effects associated with drastic dietary shifts.

Charter 2.
Evolution and The Carnivore Diet

What is the Relationship Between Evolution and the Carnivore Diet?

The carnivore diet is deeply rooted in human evolution, particularly during the Pleistocene era, also known as the Ice Age, which lasted from about 2.5 million years ago to approximately 11,700 years ago. This era overlaps almost exactly with the Paleolithic period, a time when the dietary habits of humans were shaped by the harsh climatic conditions.

During the Ice Age, the Earth's climate was significantly colder, and plant life was scarce. As a result, early humans adapted to survive by primarily consuming large, fatty animals, such as woolly mammoths, which were abundant during this time. These animals provided the necessary energy and nutrients that plants could not offer in such a cold environment.

It wasn't until the last 12,000 years, during the Neolithic period, also known as the start of the Agricultural Revolution, that humans began to include more plant foods in their diets. This shift was primarily driven by the end of the Ice Age, the extinction of many large animals, and the need for an alternative energy source.

To put this in perspective, humans have been consuming plant foods for only about 0.6% of our existence as a species, while the other 99.4% of our history was dominated by a diet rich in animal foods. This short time span is not enough for significant evolutionary changes to occur, suggesting that our bodies may still be better suited to a diet similar to that of our ancestors, which was predominantly meat-based.

Charter 3.
The Dark Side of Plant Foods

The Problem with Plant Foods
and How They Can Cause Disease
and Weight Gain

One of the primary reasons for the renewed interest in the carnivore diet is the presence of substances in plant foods that are absent in animal foods: **anti-nutrients**. Anti-nutrients are chemicals found in plants that serve as their natural defense mechanisms against bacteria, insects, and predators, including humans.

Unlike animals, which can escape predators, plants must rely on chemical defenses. Over millions of years, plants have evolved the ability to produce toxic chemicals to protect themselves from being consumed. This defense is particularly crucial for seeds, which represent the "offspring" of plants.

Anti-nutrients can adversely affect human health by reducing the body's ability to absorb essential nutrients. Some of the anti-nutrients discovered in plant foods include:

- **Glucosinolates**: Found in cruciferous vegetables like broccoli, Brussels sprouts, and cabbage, these compounds decrease iodine levels in the body.
- **Lectins**: Present in legumes (beans, peanuts, soybeans) and whole grains, lectins reduce the absorption of calcium, iron, phosphorus, and zinc. Interestingly, refined grains have lower levels of lectins compared to whole grains.

- **Phytates (Phytic Acid)**: Found in whole grains, seeds, legumes, and some nuts, phytates decrease the absorption of iron, zinc, magnesium, and calcium.
- **Amylase Inhibitors**: These are found in beans and inhibit starch digestion, which can lead to poor digestion and increase the growth of certain fungi in the gut.
- **Saponins**: Found in legumes, whole grains, and white potatoes, saponins interfere with nutrient absorption and can increase intestinal permeability, also known as "leaky gut." This condition can allow larger food molecules to enter the body, potentially triggering immune responses and leading to autoimmune conditions.
- **Oxalates**: Found in green leafy vegetables and tea, oxalates decrease calcium absorption.
- **Tannins**: Present in tea, coffee, legumes, and red wine, tannins reduce iron absorption. They are responsible for the dry feeling in your mouth after drinking red wine.
- **Trypsin Inhibitors**: Found in soybeans, these inhibitors reduce the digestion and absorption of dietary proteins.

As you can see, a wide variety of chemicals in plant foods can impact human health by affecting the body's ability to digest and absorb nutrients effectively.

Lectins, Weight Loss, and Autoimmune Conditions

Lectins, as mentioned earlier, are part of plants' natural self-defense mechanisms. Lectins are types of proteins that can bind to sugars and alter the function of those sugar molecules. Research has shown that lectins can contribute to weight gain by increasing fat storage and inducing resistance to leptin, the hormone responsible for suppressing appetite.

Leptin resistance prevents the brain from receiving the signal that the body is full, leading to increased hunger and overeating, which can result in weight gain. Additionally, lectins can attack various systems in the body, potentially contributing to chronic conditions and autoimmune disorders.

Cooking Methods
to Reduce Anti-nutrient Content

It's important to note that certain cooking methods can reduce the concentration of anti-nutrients in plant foods to some extent. This is why many cultures soak beans before cooking them, as undercooked beans can contain high levels of toxic lectins. Several instances have been reported where people were hospitalized after consuming slightly undercooked red kidney beans.

Here are some methods to reduce anti-nutrient levels:

- **Soaking**: Reduces lectin content in beans.
- **Sprouting**: Decreases the amount of anti-nutrients in seeds and legumes.
- **Fermenting**: Breaks down anti-nutrients, making the food easier to digest.
- **Boiling and Pressure Cooking**: These methods can also reduce anti-nutrient content.
- **Souring**: The process used in making sourdough bread can decrease anti-nutrient levels in grains.

Why Are Seed Oils Bad on the Carnivore Diet

Seed oils, commonly referred to as vegetable oils, are extracted from the seeds of various plants like soybeans, corn, sunflowers, safflowers, and canola (rapeseed). While these oils have become a staple in modern cooking and food production, they are generally avoided on the carnivore diet due to concerns about their high omega-6 fatty acid content and potential inflammatory effects on the body.

High Omega-6 Content and Inflammatory Effects

Omega-6 fatty acids are a type of polyunsaturated fat essential for human health. However, the modern Western diet often contains an excessive amount of omega-6 fatty acids relative to omega-3 fatty acids, leading to an imbalance that may promote inflammation. This disproportion can contribute to various chronic health issues, including heart disease, arthritis, and metabolic disorders.

Seed oils are particularly high in omega-6 fatty acids. For example:

- **Soybean oil:** Approximately 54% omega-6
- **Corn oil: Around** 57% omega-6
- **Sunflower oil:** Up to 65% omega-6
- **Safflower oil:** Approximately 75% omega-6

Consuming large quantities of these oils can disrupt the optimal omega-6 to omega-3 ratio in the body, which ideally should be close to 1:1 but in Western diets is often skewed towards 16:1 or higher. This imbalance may lead to increased production of pro-inflammatory compounds, exacerbating inflammation and potentially contributing to chronic diseases.

Processing of Seed Oils

The production of seed oils involves extensive industrial processing, which can negatively affect their nutritional quality:

1. Extraction: Seeds are cleaned and heated to high temperatures to extract the oil, a process that can cause the formation of harmful free radicals.

2. Use of Chemical Solvents: Solvents like hexane, a petroleum byproduct, are often used to maximize oil extraction. Trace amounts of these chemicals can remain in the final product.

3. Refining: The extracted oil undergoes refining processes, including bleaching and deodorizing, to improve its color and eliminate odors. These steps involve high heat and chemical additives, which can further degrade the oil's quality.

4. Hydrogenation (for some oils): Some seed oils are hydrogenated to increase shelf life and stability, leading to the creation of trans fats known to raise bad cholesterol (LDL) levels and lower good cholesterol (HDL) levels.

This intensive processing not only reduces the nutritional value of the oils but can also introduce harmful substances that may have adverse health effects when consumed regularly.

Preference for Animal Fats

The carnivore diet emphasizes whole, unprocessed animal foods, including naturally occurring animal fats such as:

- **Tallow:** Rendered beef or lamb fat
- **Lard:** Rendered pork fat
- **Butter and Ghee:** Dairy fats from cow's milk
- **Duck Fat and Other Poultry Fats**

These animal fats are predominantly saturated and monounsaturated fats, which are more stable at high cooking temperatures and less susceptible to oxidation compared to the polyunsaturated fats found in seed oils. Benefits of using animal fats include:

- **Nutrient Density:** Rich in fat-soluble vitamins A, D, E, and K2, which are essential for various bodily functions, including immune health and bone strength.

- **Improved Omega Balance:** Animal fats generally have a more favorable omega-6 to omega-3 ratio, helping to maintain a balance that may reduce inflammation.

- **Enhanced Flavor and Satiety:** Cooking with animal fats can improve the taste of foods and promote a feeling of fullness, aiding in appetite regulation.

Charter 4.
Carnivore Diet
as a Subtype of Ketogenic Diets

Carnivore Diet is a Subtype of Ketogenic Diets

The carnivore diet is essentially a subtype of the ketogenic diet. But what does this mean? Both diets share a common goal: shifting the body's primary energy source from carbohydrates to fats, leading to a metabolic state known as **ketosis**. Ketosis is the foundation of a ketogenic diet, where the body burns fat for fuel instead of carbohydrates.

In a typical ketogenic diet, carbohydrate intake is drastically reduced to less than 50 grams per day, sometimes even as low as 20 grams per day. This reduction in carbs forces the body to enter ketosis. While on a ketogenic diet, some individuals may still consume small amounts of low-sugar fruits like blueberries or raspberries, or other plant foods that contain minimal carbohydrates.

On the other hand, the carnivore diet takes this concept a step further by not only limiting carbohydrates but also eliminating all plant foods from the diet entirely. Thus, the carnivore diet can be viewed as a more restrictive form of the ketogenic diet, where the focus is solely on animal-based foods.

Interestingly, ketosis is considered our natural metabolic state. For instance, babies are born in a state of ketosis, and breastfeeding helps maintain this fat-burning state in infants. This natural inclination towards ketosis suggests that a diet like the carnivore diet may be more aligned with our biological makeup than the carbohydrate-heavy diets commonly consumed today.

Benefits of Ketosis

So, what are the benefits of shifting our main energy source away from carbohydrates and towards fats, or in other words, what are the benefits of ketosis?

One of the most significant benefits of ketosis is the facilitation of fat loss. Ketosis suppresses appetite to a much greater degree, reducing cravings and making it easier to adhere to a low-calorie diet. Additionally, ketosis leads to improved mental function, as brain cells have been shown to function better when fueled by fats rather than carbohydrates.

When following a ketogenic diet, or more specifically, a carnivore diet, blood sugar levels remain stable. This stability means that blood sugar does not drop below baseline two to three hours after a meal, as it often does on a traditional carbohydrate-heavy diet. In contrast, when consuming carbohydrates, the body secretes insulin, which causes blood sugar levels to drop, triggering hunger. By avoiding these fluctuations, the carnivore diet helps prevent frequent hunger pangs and the associated overeating.

Moreover, when the body is primarily fueled by fats, it has access to a more abundant energy source. Even in lean individuals, the body stores approximately 40,000 to 66,000 calories worth of fat, compared to only about 2,000 calories of stored carbohydrates. This means that during periods of fasting or low food intake, the body can still access its fat stores for energy, reducing the need for frequent meals.

How to Enter Ketosis

To enter a state of ketosis, you must restrict your net carbohydrate consumption to between 25 and 50 grams per day for two to three days. Net carbohydrates are calculated by subtracting the grams of fiber and sugar alcohols (such as erythritol or mannitol) from the total carbohydrates in a food item. For example, if a food contains 25 grams of carbohydrates, 5 grams of fiber, and 3 grams of sugar alcohols, the net carbohydrate content would be 17 grams.

For larger individuals, entering ketosis might be possible with an intake of up to 50 grams of net carbohydrates per day, while smaller individuals might need to reduce their intake to below 25 or even 20 grams of net carbohydrates per day to achieve ketosis.

How to Transition to a Fat-Burning Metabolism

Transitioning from a carbohydrate-based diet to a very low-carb or zero-carb diet, such as a ketogenic or carnivore diet, can sometimes lead to symptoms known as the "keto flu." This temporary condition occurs as the body adapts to using fat as its primary energy source instead of carbohydrates.

Symptoms of the keto flu can include lightheadedness, fatigue, headaches, poor concentration, and mood disturbances. These symptoms typically last for a few days to a few weeks but can be mitigated by increasing hydration and electrolyte intake (sodium, magnesium, and potassium). Consuming bone broth, which is rich in electrolytes and hydration, can also help ease this transition.

It's essential to understand that entering ketosis does not automatically mean you are fully "keto-adapted." Keto-adaptation is the process by which your body becomes more efficient at using fat as its main energy source. This adaptation can take anywhere from a few days to several weeks, depending on the individual. During this time, your body becomes more adept at burning fat for energy, leading to the long-term benefits associated with the ketogenic diet, such as weight loss and improved mental clarity.

Patience is key during this transition. While some people may feel great after just one week, others may require two to three weeks or even up to six weeks to fully adapt to a fat-burning metabolism. The rate of adaptation can vary based on genetic factors and individual metabolic responses.

Charter 5.
Meat, The Superfood!

Nutrients Found Exclusively
in Meats and Animal Foods

Meat is often considered a superfood because it is rich in several vital nutrients that are found almost exclusively in animal foods. These nutrients play essential roles in various bodily functions, particularly in energy production, anti-aging, and inflammation reduction. Below are some of the key nutrients found in meat:

Carnitine: Carnitine is crucial for fat burning as it allows the fat you consume to enter the mitochondria, where it is burned for energy. This nutrient is vital for anyone following a diet focused on fat as the primary energy source.

Carnosine: Known for its powerful anti-aging benefits, carnosine helps protect cells from oxidative stress and may reduce the risk of chronic diseases associated with aging.

Creatine: Creatine is a well-known energy source for muscles and the brain, supporting physical performance and cognitive function.

Taurine: Taurine has strong anti-inflammatory effects, which is critical because inflammation is at the root of many chronic diseases. By reducing inflammation, taurine can help lower the risk of cardiovascular diseases and other inflammatory conditions.

Retinol (Vitamin A): Retinol, the active form of vitamin A, is only found in animal foods. While plant foods contain carotenoids (precursors to vitamin A), they are not as efficiently converted to retinol in the body. Retinol is essential for vision, immune function, and skin health.

Vitamin B12: Another nutrient found exclusively in animal foods, vitamin B12 is crucial for red blood cell formation, neurological function, and DNA synthesis.

Vitamin D3: Often referred to as the sunshine vitamin, vitamin D3 is primarily obtained from exposure to sunlight. However, it is also found in certain animal foods, like wild-caught salmon. A 3-ounce filet of wild-caught salmon can provide all the vitamin D3 your body needs, while farmed salmon provides only about 25% of the recommended daily intake.

Vitamin K2: This vitamin is crucial for bone and heart health and is found exclusively in animal products. It plays a role in directing calcium to the bones and teeth, where it is needed, and away from the arteries, where it can cause harm. Vitamin K2 is distinct from vitamin K1, which is found in plant foods and has a different role in the body.

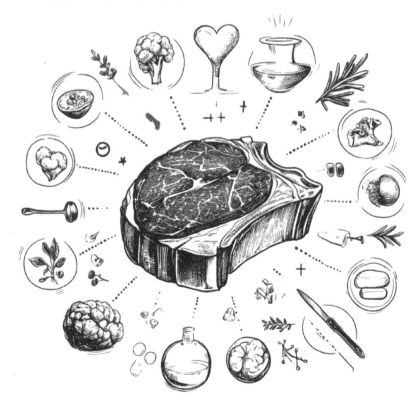

These nutrients underline the significance of meat in the human diet, particularly for those following a carnivore diet where plant-based sources of these nutrients are excluded.

Anti-aging Benefits of the Carnivore Diet

The relationship between the carnivore diet and the aging process is an important topic of discussion. It is often suggested that a high-protein diet might accelerate aging by activating a pathway known as mTOR (mammalian target of rapamycin). When mTOR is activated, it is believed to speed up the aging process.

However, what is often overlooked is the presence of carnosine in red meat and other meats, which may counteract the effects of mTOR activation. Carnosine has been shown to have potent anti-aging properties. It is believed to suppress mTOR, which could explain why carnosine is considered one of the most effective anti-aging molecules known to researchers.

Additionally, carnosine helps suppress the formation of advanced glycation end products (AGEs), which are harmful compounds formed when protein or fat combine with sugar in the bloodstream. AGEs are linked to accelerated aging and various chronic diseases. A high-sugar and high-carbohydrate diet increases the formation of AGEs, leading to damage at the cellular level and contributing to the aging process. By reducing carbohydrate intake and increasing carnosine intake through a carnivore diet, you may be able to mitigate some of these effects, promoting healthier aging.

Charter 6.
Vitamin C, Scurvy
and The Carnivore Diet

The Relationship Between Vitamin C, Carbohydrates, and Scurvy

There have been concerns regarding the potential risk of developing scurvy—a vitamin C deficiency disease—when following a carnivore diet. Typically, people obtain their vitamin C from citrus fruits or other plant-based foods that are high in this essential nutrient. Since meat generally contains lower levels of vitamin C compared to plant foods, it might seem logical to worry about deficiency.

However, among those who have been following a carnivore diet, there have been no reported cases of scurvy, even among individuals who have adhered to this diet for over 15 years without vitamin C supplementation. This raises the question: why don't carnivore diet followers develop scurvy?

Glucose   Vitamin C

One possible explanation lies in the structural similarity between glucose (a form of carbohydrate) and vitamin C. Because glucose can block the receptors for vitamin C, it prevents the full absorption of the vitamin.

The recommended daily intake of vitamin C is based on studies of people consuming a high-carbohydrate diet. Therefore, individuals on such diets might need more vitamin C because the glucose they consume interferes with the absorption of the vitamin.

In contrast, those on a low-carb or zero-carb diet, like the carnivore diet, may have a drastically reduced need for vitamin C because their receptors are no longer being blocked by glucose. Consequently, the small amounts of vitamin C found in muscle meats may be sufficient to prevent scurvy. Organ meats, which are richer in vitamin C, further reduce the risk. This might explain why people on a carnivore diet generally experience significant health improvements without the development of scurvy.

Vitamin C Content in Fresh vs. Processed Meat

There is also a distinction between the vitamin C content in fresh versus processed meat. Fresh meat does contain some vitamin C, though the amount can vary based on the type of meat and how it was raised. For example, a pound of fresh grain-fed beef contains approximately 7.24 milligrams of vitamin C, while a pound of fresh pasture-raised beef contains about 11.5 milligrams.

To prevent scurvy, the body needs around 10 milligrams of vitamin C per day. While processed meats generally have a lower vitamin C content, fresh meat consumption is typically sufficient to maintain adequate vitamin C levels. Thus, to minimize the risk of scurvy, it is advisable to focus on consuming fresh meat rather than relying heavily on processed meats like bacon.

Vitamin C and Carnitine

Another important factor to consider is the relationship between vitamin C and carnitine. Carnitine is a molecule found in abundance in animal foods, particularly in red meat. It plays a crucial role in fat metabolism by transporting fats across the mitochondrial membrane, where they can be burned for energy.

Vitamin C is required for the synthesis of carnitine in the body. However, when you consume sufficient carnitine through your diet, your body doesn't need to use its vitamin C stores to produce it. This means that a diet rich in carnitine, such as the carnivore diet, can spare your vitamin C stores, thereby reducing your need for additional vitamin C.

One of the earliest symptoms of vitamin C deficiency is fatigue, which occurs because a lack of vitamin C impairs the body's ability to produce carnitine. Without enough carnitine, the body cannot efficiently burn fat for energy. This is why individuals on a carnivore diet, which is rich in carnitine, generally do not experience scurvy or related symptoms.

For example, a 4-ounce cooked beef steak provides between 56 and 162 milligrams of carnitine, while plant foods like asparagus contain only about 0.1 milligrams per half-cup serving. This stark difference in carnitine content helps explain why vegans, who do not consume animal foods, typically have much lower carnitine levels—around 10 to 12 milligrams per day from their diet.

As a result, vegans may need to pay closer attention to their vitamin C intake, as their bodies must use more of this vitamin to synthesize the necessary carnitine. In contrast, those on a carnivore diet can maintain lower vitamin C needs due to their high dietary intake of carnitine.

Charter 7.
Transition to The Carnivore Diet

What You Need to Do to Transition Comfortably Into a Carnivore Diet

Transitioning to a carnivore diet can be a significant change, especially if you're accustomed to a diet high in carbohydrates. To make the transition as smooth and comfortable as possible, it's advisable to gradually reduce your carbohydrate intake rather than cutting them out abruptly.

If you haven't followed a low-carb diet before, start by cutting your daily carbohydrate intake in half. Continue reducing your carbohydrate consumption each day until you reach a very low-carb or zero-carb diet, which typically means consuming 20 to 30 grams of carbohydrates per day or less.

Avoid going "cold turkey." If you're currently consuming 300-400 grams of carbohydrates per day, abruptly cutting them out could lead to unpleasant side effects such as headaches, fatigue, and irritability. This isn't necessary and can be avoided with a more gradual approach.

To accurately track your carbohydrate intake, consider using tools like the USDA's FoodData Central (FDC) or apps like MyFitnessPal. These resources can help you calculate the carb content of the foods you're consuming, allowing you to make informed choices as you transition.

During the initial phase of transitioning to a carnivore diet, don't worry about being too strict with your food choices. Incorporate some low-carb options that you enjoy, such as nuts, cottage cheese sweetened with non-caloric sweeteners, or low-carb, high-protein dessert products like Halo Top ice cream or

Quest bars. These foods can help satisfy your cravings and make the transition easier by maintaining some level of dopamine and endorphin release, which are associated with pleasurable food experiences.

Once your body has adapted to a lower-carb intake, you can gradually clean up your diet by reducing or eliminating remaining plant-based foods like nuts and processed low-carb products. This approach allows for a more comfortable transition into a fat-based metabolism while still enjoying some of the foods you love.

What About Coffee/Tea?

One common question during the transition to a carnivore diet is whether you can continue drinking coffee or tea, which are plant-derived beverages. The good news is that you can generally include coffee and tea in your diet during the transition phase and even afterward, provided they don't cause any issues for you.

While these beverages contain certain plant components, they don't significantly interfere with the benefits of the carnivore diet for most people. However, if you notice that some symptoms, such as acne or autoimmune conditions, are not fully resolved on the carnivore diet, it might be worth considering eliminating coffee and tea from your diet as well. This can be done gradually as you ease into the carnivore lifestyle.

Charter 8.
Fiber, Constipation,
and The Carnivore Diet

Do You Need Fiber to Prevent Constipation?

One common misconception about the carnivore diet is that it leads to constipation due to the absence of fiber, which is exclusively found in plant foods. Public health officials and dietitians have long advocated for a high-fiber diet, emphasizing its role in preventing constipation.

Fiber is generally classified into two types: soluble and insoluble. Soluble fiber adds bulk to stools, while insoluble fiber speeds up the transit time of food through your digestive system. Together, they are believed to help prevent constipation, which is why the conventional recommendation is to consume 20 to 30 grams of fiber per day.

Given that animal foods contain no fiber, it might seem logical to assume that those following a carnivore diet would suffer from severe constipation. However, this assumption does not hold true in practice.

A study published in the *World Journal of Gastroenterology* in 2012 found that reducing fiber intake actually improved idiopathic constipation (constipation of unknown cause) in participants. More notably, those who completely eliminated fiber from their diet saw their constipation fully resolved.

This study aligns with the experiences of many carnivore diet adherents, who report that they do not suffer from constipation despite the absence of dietary fiber. It challenges the belief that fiber is essential for digestive health and suggests that reducing or eliminating it may improve bowel regularity.

Where Do People on the Carnivore Diet Get Their Fiber?

Since the carnivore diet excludes all plant foods, followers of this diet do not consume dietary fiber in the traditional sense. Instead, they rely on other mechanisms to maintain healthy digestion and prevent constipation.

One key factor is the increased intake of dietary fats, particularly saturated fats, which can have a lubricating effect on the digestive system. Fat stimulates the production of bile, which aids in the digestion of fats and can promote smoother bowel movements. Additionally, the high protein content of the diet can enhance gut motility through the action of certain amino acids that stimulate intestinal contractions.

Moreover, animal products contain connective tissues and collagen, which, while not classified as fiber, contribute to the formation of gelatinous substances when cooked. These substances can support the mucosal lining of the gut and may assist in maintaining regular digestion.

The Body's Adaptation to Low Fiber Intake

The human body is remarkably adaptable. When transitioning to a carnivore diet, the digestive system undergoes several changes to accommodate the new way of eating. Initially, some individuals may experience changes in bowel movements as the gut adjusts to the absence of fiber.

Without fiber, the body produces smaller and less frequent stools. This is not necessarily a sign of constipation but rather an indication that the body is absorbing more nutrients from the food consumed, leaving less waste to be excreted. The efficiency of nutrient absorption means there is simply less bulk moving through the intestines.

Furthermore, the reduction in fermentable fibers can lead to decreased gas production, which may alleviate bloating and discomfort associated with high-fiber diets. Some people report that their digestive systems feel more settled and less irritable without the presence of fiber.

Role of Gut Microbiota

The gut microbiota plays a crucial role in digestion, immunity, and overall health. Dietary fiber is known to feed beneficial bacteria in the gut, leading to the production of short-chain fatty acids (SCFAs) like butyrate, which have anti-inflammatory properties.

On a carnivore diet, the composition of the gut microbiota changes due to the lack of dietary fiber and the increased intake of proteins and fats. Certain bacteria that thrive on protein and fat become more prominent, while those that depend on fermentable fibers decrease.

Some may worry that the absence of fiber could negatively impact gut health. However, the body can adapt by utilizing alternative substrates for SCFA production. For instance, amino acids from dietary proteins can be fermented by specific gut bacteria to produce SCFAs. Additionally, the consumption of collagen and gelatin from animal sources may support gut lining integrity and promote a healthy mucosal barrier.

It's important to note that research on the long-term effects of a fiber-free diet on gut microbiota is still emerging. Individual responses can vary, and some people may experience digestive issues when eliminating fiber, while others may find relief from symptoms like bloating, gas, and irregular bowel movements.

Charter 9.
Health Conditions
and The Carnivore Diet

Red Meat, Heart Disease, and Cancer

There is widespread concern about the potential association between red meat consumption and an increased risk of heart disease and cancer. Many large health organizations, including the American Heart Association (AHA), have pointed to a negative relationship between red meat intake and heart health. The AHA, for example, states that red meats like beef, pork, and lamb contain higher amounts of saturated fat compared to chicken, fish, and plant-based proteins such as beans. They argue that saturated and trans fats can raise blood cholesterol levels and exacerbate heart disease.

However, recent research challenges this conventional view. A comprehensive analysis by Canberra University, involving 76 studies and more than 650,000 participants, concluded that current evidence does not clearly support the guidelines recommending low consumption of total saturated fats. Furthermore, a 2016 study emphasized that sugar, rather than saturated fat, is the primary dietary concern when it comes to increasing the risk of heart attacks.

Another prevalent concern is the belief that consuming red meat and cholesterol-rich foods, like egg yolks and shrimp, increases the risk of heart disease. This belief is rooted in the Dietary Guidelines for Americans, which historically recommended limiting dietary cholesterol intake to no more than 300 milligrams per day. Since one egg yolk contains about 200 milligrams of cholesterol, these guidelines effectively discouraged the consumption of more than one and a half egg yolks per day. However, in 2015, this recommendation was removed due to a lack of strong evidence linking dietary cholesterol with heart disease.

It's important to exercise caution if you have high blood pressure and are taking medication to manage it. When you switch to a carnivore diet or even a ketogenic diet (since the carnivore diet is a subtype of the ketogenic diet), cutting out carbohydrates can quickly normalize your blood pressure. Therefore, you should work closely with your primary care physician to adjust your blood pressure medication dosage as needed to avoid the risk of dangerously low blood pressure.

An illustrative example of the disconnect between red meat consumption and heart disease is the Maasai tribe in Kenya and northern Tanzania. The Maasai diet consists almost entirely of blood, milk, and meat, with about two-thirds of their calories coming from fat. Their cholesterol intake ranges between 600 and 2,000 milligrams per day—far exceeding past dietary recommendations. Despite their high cholesterol intake, the Maasai exhibit low blood pressure,  low overall cholesterol levels, low incidence of cholesterol gallstones, and, most notably, low rates of coronary artery disease.

Another significant concern surrounding red meat is its purported link to cancer, particularly colorectal cancer. The World Health Organization (WHO) has classified red meat as a Group 2A carcinogen, meaning it is "probably carcinogenic to humans." This classification is based on limited evidence from epidemiological studies, which show a positive association between red meat consumption and colorectal cancer, as well as strong mechanistic evidence.

However, it is crucial to recognize the limitations of these epidemiological studies. These studies often rely on large population groups and questionnaires that ask participants to recall their red meat consumption habits, which can be prone to inaccuracies. Additionally, these studies may not account for whether red meat consumption is accompanied by other unhealthy foods, such as French fries, sodas, or processed meats. For example, someone who reports eating a lot of red meat might actually be consuming it as part of fast food meals that include other unhealthy components. This can confound the results and lead to misleading conclusions.

The failure of epidemiological studies to differentiate between individuals consuming high-quality, grass-fed, organic red meat and those consuming lower-quality processed meats further complicates the issue. It is unfortunate that such studies may contribute to the stigmatization of red meat, which is one of the most nutrient-dense foods that humans have evolved to consume.

Depression, Anxiety, ADHD, Kidney Health, and Gout

Mental health conditions such as depression, anxiety, and Attention Deficit Hyperactivity Disorder (ADHD) are among the primary reasons some individuals turn to the carnivore diet. Research suggests that plant lectins—proteins found in many plant foods—can negatively impact brain cells responsible for producing dopamine, a neurotransmitter often referred to as the "happiness hormone." There is solid evidence showing that lectins can interfere with dopamine production, leading to decreased levels of this critical neurotransmitter.

When plant lectins reduce the brain's ability to produce dopamine, the result is often a diminished sense of well-being and worsening mood. By eliminating plant foods that contain these harmful lectins, the carnivore diet may help improve mood and relieve symptoms of depression, anxiety, and ADHD. Moreover, a high-protein diet associated with the carnivore lifestyle floods the brain with the precursors to dopamine and serotonin—two neurotransmitters essential for maintaining a positive mood. These precursors include the amino acids tyrosine, phenylalanine, and tryptophan, which are found in high concentrations in meat. Therefore, the more protein you consume, the more building blocks your brain has to produce dopamine and serotonin.

Another common concern is the potential impact of a high-protein diet, such as the carnivore diet, on kidney health. The fear that high protein intake may cause kidney damage is not supported by human studies. The confusion arises from the fact that protein doesn't damage healthy kidneys; rather, damaged kidneys tend to leak protein, leading to the erroneous belief that protein itself is harmful to kidney function.

There is also concern that the carnivore diet might lead to or worsen gout, a painful condition caused by the accumulation of uric acid in the joints. Gout has been historically associated with populations that consume large quantities of meat, such as the Maasai, Mongols, or Saami, who were largely unaffected by the condition. In his book "The Carnivore Diet," Dr. Shawn Baker, a 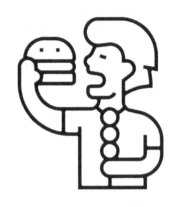 prominent advocate of the carnivore diet, notes that many of his patients have experienced improvements in or even complete resolution of gout symptoms after following the carnivore diet for a few months.

Gout is often misunderstood. It is caused by the accumulation of uric acid, and certain foods high in purines can increase uric acid production. Meat is rich in purines, which is why it is often blamed for gout. However, it is essential to understand that purines are present in most foods, and high uric acid levels do not always lead to gout. A more accurate predictor of gout risk is the consumption of sugar—particularly fructose from table sugar—and alcohol. Both sugar and alcohol can increase uric acid levels and contribute to the development of gout. Therefore, it is unnecessary to worry about red meat consumption leading to gout, especially when sugar and alcohol are the real culprits.

Binge Eating Disorder, Alcoholism, and Addiction

There is a growing body of anecdotal evidence suggesting that the carnivore diet may be effective in addressing addictive behaviors such as binge eating disorder and alcoholism. Many individuals have reported significant improvements in their relationship with food and alcohol after adopting a carnivore diet. The diet's focus on nutrient-dense, satiating animal products may help stabilize blood sugar levels and reduce cravings, which are often triggers for addictive behaviors.

For those interested in exploring this further, numerous anecdotal reports and testimonials are available online, documenting how the carnivore diet has helped individuals overcome various forms of addiction. While more scientific research is needed to fully understand the mechanisms at play, the existing evidence provides a compelling case for the potential benefits of the carnivore diet in managing and improving disordered eating and addiction.

Insulin and Recovery on the Carnivore Diet

Insulin plays a crucial role in regulating blood sugar levels by facilitating the uptake of glucose into the body's cells. Insulin sensitivity refers to how responsive cells are to insulin's signals; higher sensitivity means the body requires less insulin to process glucose. Conversely, insulin resistance can lead to elevated blood sugar levels and is a precursor to type 2 diabetes.

The carnivore diet, by eliminating carbohydrates—the primary source of glucose—can significantly impact insulin sensitivity. With a reduced intake of carbohydrates, the pancreas produces less insulin, which may improve the body's insulin response over time. Many individuals following the carnivore diet report stabilized blood sugar levels and enhanced insulin sensitivity.

Improved insulin sensitivity not only aids in blood sugar regulation but also facilitates better energy utilization and recovery after physical activity. Athletes and physically active individuals may find that the carnivore diet supports muscle recovery due to the high protein intake, which provides essential amino acids necessary for muscle repair and growth.

However, it's important to approach the diet mindfully. Drastic changes in macronutrient intake can affect hormone levels and metabolic functions. Individuals with existing insulin-related conditions should consult a healthcare professional before adopting the carnivore diet to ensure it's appropriate for their specific health needs.

Cirrhosis and the Carnivore Diet

Cirrhosis is a chronic liver disease characterized by scarring of liver tissue, leading to impaired liver function. One common concern is whether a high-protein diet like the carnivore diet is suitable for individuals with cirrhosis. Traditionally, it was believed that high protein intake could exacerbate liver problems due to the liver's role in metabolizing amino acids and producing urea.

Recent studies, however, suggest that adequate protein intake is essential for patients with liver disease to prevent muscle wasting and malnutrition. The key is to consume high-quality proteins that are easily digestible. Animal proteins, such as those emphasized in the carnivore diet, provide all essential amino acids and are considered complete proteins.

That said, those with cirrhosis must be cautious. The liver's reduced capacity to process proteins means that excessive intake could lead to an accumulation of ammonia in the blood, potentially causing hepatic encephalopathy—a decline in brain function due to liver dysfunction. Therefore, it's crucial for individuals with cirrhosis to work closely with a healthcare provider or a dietitian specialized in liver diseases to tailor the diet to their specific needs.

Moderation and medical supervision are vital. While the carnivore diet may offer benefits such as nutrient density and ease of digestion, it must be adjusted appropriately to avoid overloading the liver and to support overall health.

Ovarian Cysts and Hormonal Health

Ovarian cysts are fluid-filled sacs that can develop on or within an ovary. While many cysts are harmless and resolve on their own, some can cause discomfort or be associated with hormonal imbalances, such as those seen in Polycystic Ovary Syndrome (PCOS). PCOS is a common endocrine disorder characterized by multiple cysts on the ovaries, irregular menstrual cycles, insulin resistance, and elevated levels of androgens.

The carnivore diet may influence hormonal health through several mechanisms:

1. Insulin Regulation: By eliminating carbohydrates, the diet can stabilize blood sugar levels and improve insulin sensitivity. Improved insulin function may help reduce insulin resistance, a key factor in the development of PCOS and ovarian cysts.

2. Hormone Production: Fats and proteins are essential building blocks for hormone synthesis. The high intake of animal fats and complete proteins may support the body's production of hormones, potentially aiding in hormonal balance.

3. Inflammation Reduction: Chronic inflammation is linked to hormonal disorders. The carnivore diet's exclusion of potential inflammatory plant compounds and processed foods may reduce systemic inflammation, possibly alleviating symptoms associated with ovarian cysts.

Some women have reported improvements in menstrual regularity, reduction in cyst size, and alleviation of PCOS symptoms while following the carnivore diet. However, scientific research specifically examining the carnivore diet's effects on ovarian cysts is limited.

It's important to approach this dietary change thoughtfully:

- **Medical Consultation:** Before making significant dietary adjustments, women should consult with a gynecologist or endocrinologist to ensure the diet aligns with their health needs and to monitor hormonal levels appropriately.

- **Holistic Approach:** Diet is one aspect of managing hormonal health. Incorporating regular physical activity, stress management, and adequate sleep are also crucial components.

- **Individual Variation:** Hormonal responses can vary greatly among individuals. What works for one person may not work for another, so it's essential to pay attention to one's body and adjust as necessary.

In conclusion, while the carnivore diet may offer potential benefits for hormonal regulation and the management of ovarian cysts, more research is needed. Women considering this diet for hormonal health should do so under professional guidance to ensure safety and efficacy.

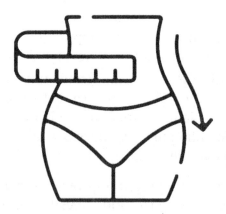

Charter 10.
Weight Loss Tips
on a Carnivore Diet

Weight Loss Tips on a Carnivore Diet

Losing weight on a carnivore diet can be achieved through several strategies that align with the principles of this diet. Below are some tips to help facilitate weight loss while following a carnivore lifestyle:

Intermittent Fasting: One effective approach is to incorporate intermittent fasting. This involves not eating breakfast until you actually feel hungry, which can help reduce overall caloric intake. During the fasting period, you can have coffee with a non-caloric sweetener or creamer to help curb hunger. Another option is bulletproof coffee, which is coffee blended with unsweetened butter. This option is preferred by many because it doesn't contain artificial sweeteners, and you can enhance its flavor with a dash of cinnamon to create a foamy, latte-like drink.

Protein to Energy Ratio (P/E Ratio): Pay attention to the protein-to-energy (P/E) ratio of the foods you consume. The P/E ratio is the amount of protein (in grams) divided by the number of calories in a food. A higher P/E ratio means the food is richer in protein relative to its caloric content. To maximize weight loss, focus on consuming leaner cuts of meat that have a high P/E ratio, as these provide ample protein while keeping calories lower.

Dealing with Carb Cravings: Cravings for carbohydrates can be challenging, especially when transitioning to a carnivore diet. A helpful strategy is to first fill up on protein. For example, you could eat fatty, satisfying meats like pulled pork or rotisserie chicken, paired with a diet soda. If you still have cravings afterward, indulge in a low-carb, high-protein treat like a 400-calorie ice cream, such as Halo Top or Eat Light. You'll often find that your urge to indulge is significantly reduced after consuming protein first.

Preventing Electrolyte Imbalances

A crucial aspect of maintaining health on a carnivore diet is managing electrolyte balance. When you cut out carbohydrates, your body's ability to retain electrolytes, particularly sodium and magnesium, decreases. This is because, in the context of a low-carbohydrate diet, your body no longer holds onto excess water and electrolytes as it would on a higher-carb diet.

To prevent symptoms like dizziness or lightheadedness, which can result from low sodium levels, it's essential to consume enough salt. Historically, tribal populations who followed a carnivorous diet would consume blood, which is rich in sodium, to remedy such symptoms. While you may not need to consume blood, increasing your salt intake is vital.

Salt and Magnesium Intake: A tablespoon of salt is approximately 40% sodium. Increasing your salt consumption not only helps with sodium balance but also improves the transport of magnesium into your cells, which is important for overall health. Adequate sodium intake can prevent hypotension (low blood pressure) and episodes of dizziness, which are more common on a zero-carb diet.

In summary, by managing your salt intake and focusing on the protein content of your meals, you can effectively support weight loss and prevent electrolyte imbalances while following a carnivore diet.

Charter 11.
Fad Diets and Notable People on The Carnivore Diet

Is The Carnivore Diet a Fad Diet?

The carnivore diet has been labeled by some as a "fad diet," a term often used to describe diets that are seen as extreme, unbalanced, or unsustainable. However, it's important to critically examine who is making these claims and what their motivations might be.

While it's true that some diets can do more harm than good and deserve the "fad" label, not all diets that differ from mainstream dietary recommendations should be dismissed as such. It's essential to recognize that many health organizations, including those that endorse certain dietary guidelines, receive funding from large food companies, which could influence their positions on what constitutes a healthy diet.

For instance, the Academy of Nutrition and Dietetics continues to recommend the daily consumption of three cups of dairy products, despite evidence suggesting a link between dairy consumption and certain cancers, such as ovarian and prostate cancer. When a diet is labeled as a "fad," it's crucial to consider the potential conflicts of interest and underlying agendas of those making the claim.

From an evolutionary perspective, the carnivore diet is far from a fad. Humans evolved during the Ice Age, a time when plant foods were scarce, and our ancestors primarily relied on meat for sustenance. If the carnivore diet were merely a fad, it wouldn't have been the diet that supported human survival and evolution for thousands of years.

In conclusion, while it's important to be cautious of diets that may be unhealthy, dismissing the carnivore diet as a fad without understanding its historical and evolutionary context is misguided. Always consider the sources of dietary advice and be aware of the potential biases that may influence their recommendations.

Notable People on The Carnivore Diet

Several notable individuals have adopted the carnivore diet and reported significant health benefits as a result. Among them is comedian Joe Rogan, who followed the carnivore diet for a month. During this time, he lost twelve pounds and experienced an improvement in his autoimmune condition, vitiligo, which causes patches of skin to lose their pigmentation. Rogan reported feeling better than ever during his time on the diet.

Psychologist Dr. Jordan Peterson is another prominent figure who has embraced the carnivore diet. On his Instagram account, @jordan.b.peterson, he shared how the diet helped him cure his lifelong depression and anxiety. Additionally, he experienced relief from numbness in his legs, a condition that had plagued him for years.

Dr. Peterson's daughter, Mikhaila Peterson, is also a well-known advocate of the carnivore diet. Her Instagram handle, @mikhailapeterson, documents her journey on the diet, which she credits with curing her lifelong depression and rheumatoid arthritis. Her arthritis was so severe that it necessitated multiple joint replacement surgeries before she turned 18. Since adopting the carnivore diet, she has experienced a significant improvement in her health and quality of life.

These personal stories highlight the potential benefits of the carnivore diet for some individuals, particularly those dealing with chronic health issues. While the diet may not be suitable for everyone, it has proven to be a transformative experience for those who have successfully adopted it.

Why Is the Carnivore Diet Criticized

The carnivore diet has attracted significant attention, both positive and negative, since its emergence into mainstream discourse. While many advocates tout its potential health benefits, the diet has also faced substantial criticism from nutritionists, medical professionals, and researchers. Understanding these criticisms is essential for anyone considering the carnivore diet, as it allows for a more informed and balanced decision.

Overview of Common Criticisms

1. Nutrient Deficiencies: Critics argue that by excluding all plant foods, the carnivore diet risks deficiencies in essential nutrients typically abundant in fruits, vegetables, and grains. These include vitamins like vitamin C and folate, minerals such as magnesium and potassium, and dietary fiber.

2. High Saturated Fat and Cholesterol Intake: A diet heavily based on animal products can lead to increased consumption of saturated fats and cholesterol. This raises concerns about the potential for elevated LDL cholesterol levels and an increased risk of heart disease.

3. Lack of Scientific Evidence: Many detractors point out that there is a lack of long-term scientific studies supporting the safety and efficacy of the carnivore diet. Most evidence is anecdotal, and rigorous clinical trials are scarce.

4. Impact on Gut Health: The absence of dietary fiber is a significant concern, as fiber is known to promote healthy digestion and support a diverse gut microbiome. A fiber-free diet may negatively affect gut bacteria balance, potentially leading to digestive issues.

5. Environmental and Ethical Concerns: Some critics highlight the environmental impact of increased meat consumption, including higher greenhouse gas emissions and resource usage.

Ethical considerations regarding animal welfare are also frequently mentioned.

6. Sustainability and Practicality: Maintaining such a restrictive diet can be challenging in social settings and may not be sustainable in the long term for many individuals.

Counterarguments and Scientific Data

1. Nutrient Intake and Bioavailability: Proponents argue that animal products contain all essential nutrients required for human health, often in more bioavailable forms. For example, vitamin B12, iron, and zinc are more readily absorbed from meat than plant sources. While vitamin C is commonly associated with fruits and vegetables, animal-sourced vitamin C is present in organ meats like liver.

2. Saturated Fat and Heart Disease: Recent studies have questioned the long-held belief that saturated fat intake directly causes heart disease. Some research suggests that the relationship between saturated fat, cholesterol levels, and heart disease is more complex than previously thought. Advocates claim that the carnivore diet can improve lipid profiles by increasing HDL ("good") cholesterol and decreasing triglycerides.

3. Emerging Research and Anecdotal Evidence: While long-term studies are limited, some clinical case reports and short-term studies have shown potential benefits of low-carbohydrate, high-fat diets on weight loss, metabolic health, and certain autoimmune conditions. The growing number of personal success stories adds to the anecdotal evidence supporting the diet.

4. Gut Health Adaptation: Supporters contend that the body can adapt to a low-fiber diet and that the gut microbiome adjusts accordingly. They argue that the reduction in fermentable fibers can decrease bloating and gastrointestinal discomfort for some individuals. Additionally, the consumption of collagen and gelatin from animal sources may support gut lining integrity.

5. Environmental Impact Nuance: Some proponents argue that sustainable farming and responsible meat sourcing can mitigate environmental concerns. They point to regenerative agriculture practices that improve soil health and sequester carbon. Moreover, they suggest that plant agriculture also has environmental costs, including deforestation and pesticide use.

6. Sustainability and Individual Variation: While the diet may be restrictive, many followers report ease of adherence due to simplified meal planning and reduced cravings. The sustainability of the diet can vary among individuals, and some may adopt a more flexible "carnivore-ish" approach to suit their lifestyle.

Encouraging Informed Decision-Making

Making an informed choice about adopting the carnivore diet involves careful consideration of both the potential benefits and drawbacks. Here are some recommendations for those contemplating this dietary approach:

- **Consult Healthcare Professionals:** Before making significant dietary changes, especially those as drastic as the carnivore diet, consult with a healthcare provider or a registered dietitian. They can help assess your individual health needs and monitor any changes.

- **Personalize the Approach:** Recognize that dietary needs are highly individual. What works for one person may not work for another. Consider starting with a less restrictive version of the diet and adjust based on your body's responses.

- **Monitor Health Markers:** Regularly track important health markers such as blood pressure, lipid profiles, and nutrient levels. This monitoring can help identify any adverse effects early on.

- **Stay Informed with Current Research:** Nutrition science is continually evolving. Stay updated with the latest research findings to make evidence-based decisions about your diet.

- **Consider Ethical and Environmental Factors:** Reflect on how your food choices align with your values regarding animal welfare and environmental sustainability. If these are concerns, explore options like sourcing meat from ethical and sustainable farms.

- **Listen to Your Body:** Pay attention to how you feel on the diet. Increased energy levels, improved mood, and better digestion are positive signs, whereas persistent fatigue, digestive issues, or other negative symptoms may indicate that adjustments are needed.

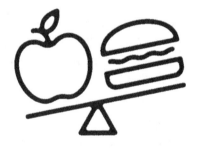

Charter 12.
Sample Meal Plan
on The Carnivore Diet

Meal Plan and Foods to Eat on a Carnivore Diet

A sample meal plan on the carnivore diet can provide you with a variety of nutrient-dense options while ensuring that you stick to the principles of this diet. Here's what a typical day might look like:

For Breakfast

- **Eggs and Bacon:** A classic option that's both filling and high in protein. If you're transitioning or not adhering strictly to the carnivore diet, you could also add cheese to this meal.

- **Eggs and Sausage:** Another savory choice that pairs well with coffee. If you prefer, you can add a creamer or artificial sweetener to your coffee. Alternatively, try blending your coffee with unsweetened butter (commonly known as bulletproof coffee), which provides a creamy, satisfying start to your day.

- **Eggs and Steak:** A heartier breakfast option that ensures you're getting plenty of protein early in the day.

For Lunch

- **Ribeye Steak:** This cut of meat is one of the fattiest and most flavorful. It's perfect for those who aren't concerned with cutting calories.

- **Tenderloin Steak:** If you're focusing on reducing body fat, opt for a leaner cut like tenderloin steak. You could pair this with salmon for added variety.
- **Cod Fish with Pulled Pork:** This combination offers a mix of lean protein and savory pork.
- **Lobster and Shrimp with Garlic Butter:** A more luxurious lunch option that's both delicious and entirely carnivore-compliant.

For Dinner
- **Rotisserie Chicken and Ground Turkey:** A satisfying and versatile meal that's easy to prepare.
- **Burger Patty with Cheese:** A simple yet delicious option. You can add diced onions as a garnish if desired.
- **Ground Beef with Garnishes:** Ground beef is a staple on the carnivore diet. Topping it with cheese or onions can add flavor and variety.

Additional Foods
- **Grilled Chicken Breasts:** Especially good if you're focusing on reducing body fat.
- **Rotisserie Chicken with Skin:** Higher in fat but incredibly flavorful. It's a great option if you're not worried about cutting calories.
- **Chicken Wings and Thighs:** Perfect for those who enjoy richer, fattier cuts of meat.
- **Seafood:** Shrimp, salmon, seared tuna, sushi, lobster, crab meat, white fish like tilapia or cod, and even octopus are all excellent choices on the carnivore diet.
- **Ground Beef or Turkey Patties:** These can be topped with melted cheese for a quick and easy meal. They're also a convenient option if you're eating out at a fast-food restaurant—just order a bunless burger topped with cheese.

The variety of options available on the carnivore diet ensures that you can enjoy flavorful, satisfying meals while adhering to the dietary guidelines. The key is to focus on high-quality animal products that provide the nutrients your body needs.

30-DAY

CARNIVORE DIET

MEAL PLAN

WEEK 1

Day 1

Breakfast: Steak and Eggs
Lunch: Grilled Chicken Skewers
Dinner: Ribeye Steak with Garlic Butter

Day 2

Breakfast: Omelette with Cheddar Cheese
Lunch: Ground Beef Carnivore Chili
Dinner: Roast Chicken with Herb Butter

Day 3

Breakfast: Carnivore Pancakes (Egg and Pork Rinds)
Lunch: Bacon-Wrapped Chicken Breasts
Dinner: Grilled Lamb Chops

Day 4

Breakfast: Sausage & Cheese Breakfast Casserole
Lunch: Chicken Alfredo (Carnivore Style)
Dinner: Grilled T-Bone Steak

Day 5

Breakfast: Smoked Salmon and Scrambled Eggs
Lunch: Garlic Shrimp Scampi
Dinner: Beef Tenderloin with Blue Cheese Crust

Day 6

Breakfast: Egg Muffins with Sausage
Lunch: Beef and Lamb Meatloaf
Dinner: Grilled Ribeye Steak with Rosemary Butter

Day 7

Breakfast: Breakfast Egg & Ham Bake
Lunch: Grilled Chicken Wings
Dinner: Braised Short Ribs

WEEK 2

Day 8

Breakfast: Poached Eggs
Lunch: Shrimp and Crab Boil
Dinner: Lamb Shoulder Roast

Day 9

Breakfast: Soft-Boiled Eggs with Sea Salt
Lunch: Turkey Drumsticks with Garlic Butter
Dinner: Garlic Herb Prime Rib

Day 10

Breakfast: Meat Lover's Breakfast Skillet (Bacon, Sausage, Eggs)
Lunch: Stuffed Turkey Thighs
Dinner: Smoked Beef Ribs

Day 11

Breakfast: Cream Cheese and Egg Puffs
Lunch: Grilled Chicken Skewers
Dinner: Chuck Roast with Bone Broth Gravy

Day 12

Breakfast: Eggs Benedict with Hollandaise Sauce
Lunch: Crab Cakes (Carnivore Style)
Dinner: Duck Breast with Crispy Skin

Day 13

Breakfast: Bone Broth Breakfast Soup
Lunch: Chicken Thighs in Cream Sauce
Dinner: Grilled T-Bone Steak

Day 14

Breakfast: Carnivore Breakfast Pizza (Eggs, Bacon, Cheese)
Lunch: Blackened Catfish
Dinner: Veal Cutlets with Lemon Butter Sauce

WEEK 3

Day 15

Breakfast: Scrambled Eggs with Bacon Bits
Lunch: BBQ Chicken Drumsticks
Dinner: Braised Short Ribs

Day 16

Breakfast: Omelette with Cheddar Cheese
Lunch: Crispy Pork Belly Bites
Dinner: Grilled Ribeye Steak with Garlic Butter

Day 17

Breakfast: Carnivore Pancakes (Egg and Pork Rinds)
Lunch: Garlic Shrimp Scampi
Dinner: Roast Chicken with Herb Butter

Day 18

Breakfast: Egg Muffins with Sausage
Lunch: Ground Beef Carnivore Chili
Dinner: Lamb Shoulder Roast

Day 19

Breakfast: Steak and Eggs

Lunch: Grilled Chicken Wings

Dinner: Beef and Lamb Meatloaf

Day 20

Breakfast: Sausage & Cheese Breakfast Casserole

Lunch: Bacon-Wrapped Chicken Breasts

Dinner: Grilled T-Bone Steak

Day 21

Breakfast: Smoked Salmon and Scrambled Eggs

Lunch: Shrimp and Crab Boil

Dinner: Garlic Herb Prime Rib

WEEK 4

Day 22

Breakfast: Poached Eggs

Lunch: Chicken Alfredo (Carnivore Style)

Dinner: Beef Tenderloin with Blue Cheese Crust

Day 23

Breakfast: Soft-Boiled Eggs with Sea Salt

Lunch: Stuffed Turkey Thighs

Dinner: Smoked Beef Ribs

Day 24

Breakfast: Meat Lover's Breakfast Skillet (Bacon, Sausage, Eggs)

Lunch: Grilled Chicken Skewers

Dinner: Chuck Roast with Bone Broth Gravy

Day 25

Breakfast: Cream Cheese and Egg Puffs
Lunch: Crab Cakes (Carnivore Style)
Dinner: Duck Breast with Crispy Skin

Day 26

Breakfast: Eggs Benedict with Hollandaise Sauce
Lunch: Chicken Thighs in Cream Sauce
Dinner: Grilled Lamb Chops

Day 27

Breakfast: Bone Broth Breakfast Soup
Lunch: Blackened Catfish
Dinner: Veal Cutlets with Lemon Butter Sauce

Day 28

Breakfast: Carnivore Breakfast Pizza (Eggs, Bacon, Cheese)
Lunch: BBQ Chicken Drumsticks
Dinner: Braised Short Ribs
Week 5

Day 29

Breakfast: Scrambled Eggs with Bacon Bits
Lunch: Crispy Pork Belly Bites
Dinner: Grilled Ribeye Steak with Rosemary Butter

Day 30

Breakfast: Omelette with Cheddar Cheese
Lunch: Garlic Shrimp Scampi
Dinner: Roast Chicken with Herb Butter

Charter 13.
Calculate Your Daily Calorie Goal to Reach Your Fitness Goals

To achieve your fitness goals, whether it's maintaining your current weight, losing body fat, or gaining muscle, accurately calculating your daily caloric needs is essential. The key to this calculation is understanding your Basal Metabolic Rate (BMR) and Total Energy Expenditure (TEE).

Step 1: Calculate Your Basal Metabolic Rate (BMR)

Your BMR represents the number of calories your body requires to function at rest. The Mifflin-St. Jeor Equation, simplified for use with U.S. customary measurements, is:

For Males:

BMR=4.54×weight in lbs+15.88×height in inches−5×age in years+5

For Females:

BMR=4.54×weight in lbs+15.88×height in inches−5×age in years−161

Why Are These Factors Used?

These simplified formulas use coefficients that incorporate the necessary conversions from the metric system. The Mifflin-St. Jeor Equation was originally developed to use kilograms for weight and centimeters for height, which are standard in the metric system.

- **Weight Conversion:** The factor 4.54 replaces the original metric-based factor (10/2.205), allowing you to input weight directly in pounds. This adjustment is necessary because the original formula uses kilograms, so we divide the weight in pounds by 2.205 to convert it to kilograms within the equation.
- **Height Conversion:** The factor 15.88 replaces the original metric-based factor (6.25 × 2.54), allowing you to input height directly in inches. The original formula uses centimeters, so we multiply the height in inches by 2.54 to convert it to centimeters within the equation.

These adjusted coefficients allow you to calculate your BMR without having to manually convert pounds to kilograms or inches to centimeters, making the formula easier to use with U.S. customary measurements.

Step 2: Adjust for Physical Activity

After calculating your BMR, you need to factor in your daily physical activity to determine your Total Energy Expenditure (TEE). Multiply your BMR by a physical activity factor that reflects your lifestyle:

- **Sedentary (little or no exercise):** 1.2
- **Lightly active (light exercise/sports 1–3 days/week):** 1.375
- **Moderately active (moderate exercise/sports 3–5 days/week):** 1.55
- **Very active (hard exercise/sports 6–7 days/week):** 1.725
- **Strenuous work or highly active leisure time:** 2.0–2.4

This final number represents your TEE, which is the total number of calories you need to consume daily to maintain your current weight.

Step 3: Adjust Caloric Intake Based on Your Goals

- **To Maintain Weight:** Consume the exact number of calories as your TEE.
- **To Lose Weight:** Create a caloric deficit by subtracting approximately 500 calories from your TEE. This should lead to a loss of about one pound of body fat per week, as one pound of body fat equals 3,500 calories.
- **To Gain Muscle:** Add a small number of calories to your TEE (about 60 calories for men, 30 calories for women), or at the very least, avoid creating a caloric deficit.

Quick Estimation Method

If you're in a hurry, you can quickly estimate your daily caloric needs using the same simplified Mifflin-St. Jeor equation and activity factors. For instance:

For Sedentary Lifestyle: Multiply your BMR by 1.2.

For Moderately Active Lifestyle: Multiply your BMR by 1.55.

By following these steps, you can determine your daily caloric needs more accurately and tailor your diet to meet your fitness goals, whether it's maintaining your current physique, losing weight, or gaining muscle mass.

Adapting the Carnivore Diet for Fitness Goals

The carnivore diet can be tailored to meet your specific fitness objectives:

- **For Weight Loss:**

1. Focus on lean cuts of meat to reduce caloric intake while still feeling satiated.

2. Prioritize high-protein foods, as protein increases satiety and has a higher thermic effect, meaning your body uses more energy to digest it.

- **For Muscle Gain:**

  1. Include fattier cuts of meat to increase caloric intake.

  2. Ensure adequate protein consumption to support muscle repair and growth.

  3. Incorporate organ meats for additional nutrients like iron and B vitamins.

- **For Maintenance:**

  1. Balance your intake of lean and fatty meats to meet your caloric needs without significant deficits or surpluses.

  2. Listen to your body's hunger cues to maintain energy balance.

Additional Tips for Success

1. Tracking Progress

- **Keep a Food Journal:** Document what you eat to monitor caloric intake and nutrient composition.
- **Measure Physical Changes:** Use a combination of weight tracking, body measurements, and progress photos.
- **Adjust as Needed:** If you're not seeing the desired results, reassess your caloric intake and activity levels.

2. Importance of Recovery and Sleep

- **Adequate Sleep:** Aim for 7–9 hours of quality sleep per night to support muscle recovery, hormonal balance, and overall health.
- **Rest Days:** Incorporate rest days into your exercise routine to prevent overtraining and reduce the risk of injury.
- **Stress Management:** Practice relaxation techniques like deep breathing, meditation, or yoga to reduce cortisol levels, which can impact weight and muscle gain.

3. Pre- and Post-Workout Nutrition on the Carnivore Diet

- **Pre-Workout:**

1). Consume easily digestible proteins like eggs or lean meats 1–2 hours before exercise to provide amino acids for muscle fuel.

2). Stay hydrated to optimize performance.

- **Post-Workout:**

1). Prioritize protein-rich foods within 30–60 minutes after exercise to aid muscle recovery.

2). Include sources of healthy fats to support overall calorie intake and nutrient absorption.

4. Hydration and Electrolytes

- **Stay Hydrated:** Drink plenty of water throughout the day, as high-protein diets can increase water needs.

- **Electrolyte Balance:**

Sodium: Essential for nerve function and muscle contractions. Consider adding a pinch of salt to your water or meals.

Potassium and Magnesium: Important for heart health and muscle function. While these are less abundant in animal products, they can be found in meats like beef and pork.

Supplementation: If necessary, use electrolyte supplements approved for the carnivore diet to maintain proper levels.

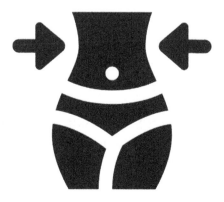

Charter 14.
Supplements
and Nutrient Optimization

Achieving optimal health on the carnivore diet involves more than just consuming animal products; it also requires attention to micronutrient intake. While animal foods are rich in many essential nutrients, there are certain vitamins and minerals that may require additional consideration. This chapter explores the role of trace minerals like boron, discusses whether supplementation is necessary, and provides guidance on optimizing nutrient intake while following the carnivore diet.

Do You Need Boron on the Carnivore Diet?

Role of Trace Minerals

Boron is a trace mineral found in various foods, particularly fruits, vegetables, nuts, and legumes. Although not officially classified as an essential nutrient, boron plays a role in several bodily functions:

Bone Health: Boron is believed to influence the metabolism of minerals involved in bone development, such as calcium, magnesium, and vitamin D. It may help improve bone density and reduce the risk of osteoporosis.

Hormonal Regulation: Some studies suggest that boron can impact the body's production and utilization of hormones like estrogen and testosterone, potentially affecting muscle mass and cognitive function.

Inflammation and Oxidative Stress: Boron may exhibit anti-inflammatory properties and help combat oxidative stress by influencing antioxidant enzymes.

How to Obtain Necessary Nutrients Through Diet

On the carnivore diet, the intake of boron is naturally low due to the exclusion of plant foods where boron is most abundant. However, it's important to consider whether this poses a significant concern.

Do You Need to Supplement Boron?

Given that boron is not classified as an essential nutrient and the body requires it only in trace amounts, most individuals on the carnivore diet may not need to supplement it. The human body can function properly without high boron intake, and deficiency symptoms are rare and not well-defined.

Alternative Sources of Boron

While boron is scarce in animal products, some sources suggest that trace amounts might be present in certain animal tissues due to the animals' consumption of boron-containing plants. However, these amounts are likely minimal.

Balancing Trace Minerals

Focusing on a varied intake of animal foods can help ensure that you're getting a broad spectrum of nutrients:

Organ Meats: Liver, kidney, and heart are nutrient-dense and provide vitamins and minerals not abundantly found in muscle meats.

Bone Broth: Rich in minerals like calcium, magnesium, phosphorus, and trace elements that support bone health.

Seafood: Fish and shellfish offer iodine, selenium, zinc, and omega-3 fatty acids, contributing to overall mineral balance.

What Is the Best Supplement to Take on the Carnivore Diet?

While the carnivore diet supplies many essential nutrients, certain vitamins and minerals may be lacking or require special attention. Supplementation can help fill these gaps to ensure optimal health.

Recommendations for Essential Supplements

1. Electrolytes

Sodium: Necessary for nerve function and fluid balance. Increased intake may be required, as low-carb diets can cause the body to excrete more sodium.

Recommendation: Add salt to your meals or drink salted water to maintain adequate sodium levels.

Potassium: Supports muscle contractions and heart function. While meat contains potassium, intake might be insufficient for some individuals.

Recommendation: Include potassium-rich animal foods like red meat and fish. In some cases, supplementation may be considered under professional guidance.

Magnesium: Involved in over 300 enzymatic reactions, including energy production and muscle function.

Recommendation: Consume foods like bone broth and fatty fish. If symptoms of deficiency arise (muscle cramps, sleep disturbances), a magnesium supplement may be beneficial.

2. Vitamin D

Role: Essential for bone health, immune function, and inflammation regulation.

Sources: Fatty fish (salmon, mackerel), egg yolks, and liver provide vitamin D, but sunlight exposure is also crucial.

Recommendation: Aim for regular sunlight exposure. In regions with limited sunlight, consider vitamin D supplementation after consulting with a healthcare provider.

3. Vitamin K2

Role: Works synergistically with vitamin D to regulate calcium metabolism, supporting bone and cardiovascular health.

Sources: Found in animal products like liver, egg yolks, and certain cheeses.

Recommendation: Incorporate these foods into your diet regularly.

4. Omega-3 Fatty Acids

Role: Support heart health, reduce inflammation, and promote brain function.

Sources: Fatty fish such as salmon, sardines, and mackerel.

Recommendation: Consume fatty fish several times a week or consider a high-quality fish oil supplement.

Vitamin Deficiencies to Watch For

1. Vitamin C

Concern: Vitamin C is typically associated with fruits and vegetables. Deficiency can lead to scurvy, characterized by fatigue, gum disease, and skin issues.

Counterpoints

Reduced Requirement: Some proponents argue that low-carb diets reduce the body's need for vitamin C due to decreased glucose competition for cellular uptake.

Animal Sources: Small amounts of vitamin C are present in raw liver and other organ meats.

Recommendation: While deficiency is rare among carnivore dieters, if concerned, include organ meats in your diet. If symptoms of deficiency appear, consult a healthcare professional.

2. Folate (Vitamin B9)

Role: Important for DNA synthesis and repair, red blood cell formation, and fetal development during pregnancy.

Sources: Liver is an excellent source of folate.

Recommendation: Include liver in your diet, especially for women of childbearing age.

3. Fiber

Concern: Lack of dietary fiber may impact gut health.

Counterpoints

Adaptation: The body may adapt to a low-fiber diet without adverse effects on bowel movements.

Gut Microbiota: Changes in gut bacteria composition may occur, but the long-term implications are still under research.

Recommendation: Monitor digestive health and consult a professional if issues arise.

4. Iodine

Role: Essential for thyroid function.

Sources: Seafood and iodized salt.

Recommendation: Include seafood in your diet and use iodized salt if necessary.

Charter 15.
Lifestyle Factors

Is Sunscreen Safe on the Carnivore Diet?

The carnivore diet focuses on consuming only animal-based foods, but its principles can extend beyond nutrition to other aspects of lifestyle, including the products we apply to our bodies. One question that arises is whether sunscreen is safe or compatible with the carnivore lifestyle, especially considering the chemicals present in many skincare products.

Discussion of Chemicals in Skincare Products

Many commercial sunscreens contain a variety of synthetic chemicals designed to block or absorb ultraviolet (UV) radiation from the sun. Some of the common active ingredients include oxybenzone, octinoxate, avobenzone, and homosalate. These compounds have raised concerns due to their potential hormonal disruption, skin irritation, and environmental impact.

Oxybenzone, for example, is a chemical filter that absorbs UV light but has been shown to penetrate the skin and enter the bloodstream. Studies suggest that it may have estrogenic effects, potentially disrupting endocrine function. Additionally, these chemicals can contribute to coral reef bleaching when washed off in the ocean, posing environmental hazards.

From a carnivore lifestyle perspective, which emphasizes natural and ancestral living, applying synthetic chemicals to the skin may contradict the philosophy of reducing exposure to potentially harmful substances.

Natural Alternatives and Overall Skin Health

To align with the carnivore lifestyle and minimize exposure to synthetic chemicals, consider using natural sunscreen alternatives:

- **Mineral Sunscreens:** Products containing zinc oxide or titanium dioxide act as physical barriers that reflect UV rays. They are generally recognized as safe and effective, with minimal skin penetration.
- **Natural Oils with Low SPF:** Some natural oils like coconut oil, red raspberry seed oil, and carrot seed oil offer minimal sun protection (SPF 4–7). While they are not sufficient for prolonged sun exposure, they can provide a light barrier for short periods outdoors.
- **Protective Clothing:** Wearing hats, sunglasses, and clothing that covers the skin can physically block UV rays without the need for topical products.
- **Gradual Sun Exposure:** Building up sun exposure gradually can enhance the skin's natural tolerance. Starting with short periods in the sun and increasing over time can stimulate melanin production, providing some natural protection.

Overall Skin Health

Consuming a nutrient-dense carnivore diet can contribute to healthier skin from the inside out. High intake of vitamins A, D, E, and K2, along with essential fatty acids, supports skin integrity and may improve the skin's resilience to sun exposure.

Impact of Lifestyle on Diet Success

While diet plays a crucial role in health, other lifestyle factors significantly influence the success of the carnivore diet and overall well-being.

Stress Management

Chronic stress can undermine health by elevating cortisol levels, leading to inflammation, hormonal imbalances, and impaired immune function. Incorporating stress-reduction techniques is essential:

- **Mindfulness and Meditation:** Practicing mindfulness can help reduce anxiety and promote mental clarity.
- **Breathing Exercises:** Techniques like deep breathing or the 4-7-8 method can activate the parasympathetic nervous system, promoting relaxation.
- **Time in Nature:** Spending time outdoors can reduce stress levels and improve mood.

Physical Activity

Regular physical activity complements the carnivore diet by enhancing metabolic health, supporting muscle growth, and improving cardiovascular function.

- **Strength Training:** Builds muscle mass and bone density, aiding in weight management and metabolic rate.
- **Aerobic Exercise:** Activities like walking, running, or swimming improve cardiovascular health and endurance.
- **Flexibility and Mobility:** Practices like yoga or stretching enhance joint health and reduce injury risk.

Sleep and Recovery

Adequate sleep is vital for hormonal balance, cognitive function, and physical recovery.

- **Aim for 7–9 Hours:** Most adults need between seven and nine hours of sleep per night for optimal health.
- **Establish a Routine:** Going to bed and waking up at consistent times helps regulate the body's internal clock.
- **Sleep Environment:** Ensure your bedroom is dark, quiet, and cool to promote restful sleep.

Conclusion

As we reach the culmination of this exploration into the carnivore diet, it's evident that this way of eating offers a unique and powerful approach to reclaiming health and vitality through simplicity. By focusing on nutrient-rich, animal-based foods, you're embracing a diet that has sustained humans for millennia, aligning closely with our evolutionary heritage.

Summing Up

Throughout this book, we've delved into the foundational aspects of the carnivore diet, from its historical roots and evolutionary significance to the practical steps for implementing it in your daily life. We've examined the potential pitfalls of plant-based anti-nutrients, the importance of nutrient optimization, and how to tailor the diet to achieve your specific fitness goals.

The potential benefits are significant—improved energy levels, enhanced mental clarity, weight management, and relief from chronic health conditions. Personal stories from notable individuals have highlighted the transformative impact this diet can have, offering inspiration and real-world evidence of its effectiveness.

Importance of Individual Approach

It's crucial to recognize that everyone's body is unique. What works wonders for one person may not yield the same results for another. Factors such as genetics, lifestyle, existing health conditions, and personal preferences play significant roles in how you might respond to the carnivore diet.

We encourage you to listen to your body and be attentive to how you feel as you make dietary changes. Adjustments may be necessary to suit your individual needs, whether that's tweaking macronutrient ratios, incorporating specific supplements, or modifying meal timing and portion sizes. Remember, the goal is not just to follow a diet but to cultivate a sustainable lifestyle that promotes your overall well-being.

Encouraging Professional Consultations

While the information provided in this book offers a comprehensive guide to the carnivore diet, it's important to involve healthcare professionals in your journey. Consulting with a qualified healthcare provider or a registered dietitian can offer personalized advice, help monitor your progress, and ensure that your approach is safe and effective.

Professional guidance is especially important if you have pre-existing health conditions such as diabetes, heart disease, kidney issues, or if you're pregnant or nursing. A healthcare professional can assist in:

- **Evaluating Your Health Status:** Assessing baseline health markers to tailor the diet to your needs.
- **Monitoring Nutrient Levels:** Ensuring you're obtaining all essential vitamins and minerals.
- **Adjusting Medications:** Modifying any medications that may be affected by dietary changes.
- **Providing Support:** Offering encouragement and strategies to overcome challenges.

By collaborating with professionals, you can optimize the benefits of the carnivore diet while minimizing potential risks.

Final Thoughts

Embarking on the carnivore diet is more than changing what's on your plate—it's a holistic shift towards embracing simplicity, ancestral wisdom, and a focus on nourishing your body with whole, unprocessed foods. This journey is an opportunity to reconnect with natural eating patterns, improve your health, and enhance your quality of life.

We encourage you to take what you've learned and apply it with enthusiasm and mindfulness. Experiment with different foods, listen to your body's signals, and make adjustments as needed. Stay informed by keeping up with the latest research and consider joining communities of like-minded individuals for support and shared experiences.

Remember, every step you take towards embracing the carnivore diet is a step towards a healthier, more vibrant you. We wish you success and joy on your journey. Stay curious, stay committed, and enjoy the profound simplicity and power of this way of eating.

Appendices

Personal Stories and Testimonials

I've been following the carnivore diet for just a week now, so I'm still in the adaptation phase. Here's what I've experienced so far:

The withdrawal from carbs mainly involves irritability and intense cravings for sugar and carbohydrates. It's a dopamine response and isn't directly related to the carnivore diet itself. These feelings should subside over time because carbs act like pure dopamine—in fact, many products and services in the U.S. are designed to trigger that response. Addiction is profitable, after all. Also, carbs function similarly to opioids (not directly, but the glucose they convert into does), so you're essentially going through a mild form of opioid withdrawal. It's tough, I get it. But should our food really act like a drug? I don't think so.

Regarding nutrient deficiencies, I've finally figured out a plan. I'm incorporating MCT oil as my body adjusts to using ketones for energy—yes, it's not strictly carnivore, but it's a temporary aid. I'm also paying attention to electrolytes since I'm flushing out retained water, and adding extra salt helps with that. For a natural multivitamin, I'm including liver in my diet. I'm still fine-tuning things like collagen powder. Getting as much sunlight as possible is important too, since sunlight helps convert cholesterol into Vitamin D, which can help keep cholesterol levels down.

My daily meals are pretty straightforward: sardines, which have a 1:1 or even 1.5:1 fat-to-protein ratio if not just relying on beef; a few soft-boiled eggs each day; and extra butter for additional energy. I keep it simple calorie-wise, consuming about a pound of beef per day—I'm a 115-pound female.

Benefits I've noticed so far:

- **Digestive Relief:** All my gastrointestinal distress has completely vanished. I tested this by eating a little bread, and it made my body feel terrible. That stuff is bad news for me—I now know I can't tolerate any bread at all.

- **Mental Clarity:** My focus has sharpened, my mood is more stable, the brain fog has lifted, and I feel a higher sense of empathy. I'm better at handling stress and adapting to changes. I'm less resistant to doing chores and have more motivation overall—just a greater sense of peace.

- **Steady Energy:** I have more energy that's consistent throughout the day, even when I'm hungry.

- **Changed Hunger Cues:** Hunger feels different now—it's more of a gentle awareness rather than that ravenous, irritable feeling. It's more intuitive and takes a bit of time to recognize.

- **Reduced Pain:** I have nerve damage in my wrist, and the pain has significantly decreased (though it would be even better if it were arthritis-related, but my issue is from trauma, not autoimmune).

- **No More Migraines:** Finally, I don't suffer from debilitating migraines anymore.

- **Improved Ear Symptoms:** Symptoms of Ménière's disease like tinnitus, ear fullness, vertigo, and hearing loss are diminishing.

- **Enhanced Senses:** My eyesight and hearing have improved, and all my senses seem sharper.

- **Muscle Gain:** I've gained a noticeable amount of muscle without working out—I even have strong (though not visibly defined) abs now! Walking and physical activities feel much easier.

On the other hand, my boyfriend isn't taking the diet as seriously and is now complaining about how much he's suffering. It's easy to mess up any diet if it's done lazily or half-heartedly. I'd be cautious about listening to people who don't follow it properly and then criticize the diet. Like any dietary approach, the carnivore diet works well if done correctly. If someone goes vegan (which

I don't recommend) and eats only french fries and ketchup, of course they'll feel awful. The same goes for the carnivore diet if all you consume is ground beef without considering other nutritional needs like hydration.

Story 2

I gave the carnivore diet a try and felt absolutely fantastic. Between August 9th and August 30th, 2016, I ate exclusively meat, eggs, and cheese at every meal. My breakfasts could include as many as 12 eggs and 8 to 10 beef patties or sausages. I'd do the same for lunch—I was staying in a motel with an open breakfast bar, so I'd stock up for both breakfast and lunch. For dinner, I'd have an Atkins shake. In total, I was consuming between 3,000 and 4,000 calories a day.

Initially, I didn't see much weight loss, but I felt incredible. Then I learned that your body can temporarily replace fat in your fat cells with water. Before long, I started experiencing what's known as a "whoosh" effect—the weight began to drop rapidly, almost a pound a day. Over 90 days, I went from 219 pounds down to 148 pounds.

As I progressed, I transitioned to an intermittent fasting regimen, where I continued to eat plenty of meat for calories and added vegetables to help with digestion. This approach worked extremely well. While the meat might not have been the sole factor in my weight loss, it helped me feel satisfied and not deprived or restricted. I'm still following this dietary pattern and continue to see excellent progress and maintain my results.

Story 3

I decided to embark on the carnivore diet three months ago, curious about how it might impact my health and well-being. Prior to this, I struggled with persistent fatigue, joint pain, and stubborn weight that just wouldn't budge despite trying various diets and exercise routines.

The first couple of weeks were challenging. I experienced what's often called the "keto flu"—headaches, low energy, and irritability—as my body adjusted to the absence of carbohydrates.

But I stayed committed, focusing on eating a variety of meats, including beef, chicken, fish, and incorporating organ meats like liver for their rich nutrient content. I also made sure to include plenty of natural fats from butter and bone marrow to keep my energy levels up.

As I moved into the third week, I started noticing significant changes:

- **Increased Energy:** The fatigue that had been my constant companion began to fade. I woke up feeling refreshed and sustained that energy throughout the day without the usual afternoon slump.

- **Weight Loss:** The scale started moving in the right direction. Over the past three months, I've lost a total of 25 pounds. More importantly, I feel lighter and more comfortable in my body.

- **Reduced Joint Pain:** The aches in my knees and ankles diminished substantially. Activities like walking up stairs or going for a jog no longer felt like a chore.

- **Improved Digestion:** Bloating and indigestion became things of the past. My digestion feels more regular and predictable now.

- **Mental Clarity:** Perhaps one of the most surprising benefits has been the improvement in my mental clarity. The brain fog lifted, and I found myself more focused and productive at work.

- **Better Sleep:** My sleep quality improved dramatically. I fall asleep faster and wake up less frequently during the night.

Social situations were initially tricky. Friends and family were skeptical, often questioning the healthfulness of such a restrictive diet. However, as they observed the positive changes in me, some became curious and even supportive. I've learned to navigate restaurant menus by opting for steak, burgers without the bun, or grilled fish, which makes dining out manageable.

I also paid close attention to hydration and electrolyte balance, adding a pinch of salt to my water and occasionally drinking bone broth to ensure I was getting enough sodium and potassium.

This journey hasn't been without its challenges, but the benefits I've experienced make it worthwhile. I plan to continue with the carnivore diet, possibly introducing some low-carb vegetables in the future to see how my body responds. For now, I'm grateful for the improvements in my health and excited to see where this path leads me.

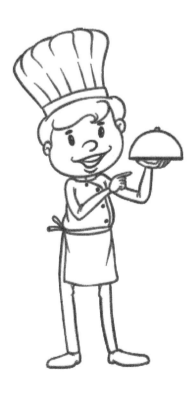

CARNIVORE DIET RECIPE

Breakfast

Breakfast Egg & Ham Bake

Ingredients:
- 6 large eggs
- 12 slices ham
- 1/2 cup heavy cream
- 1 tbsp Dijon mustard
- 1 tbsp fresh thyme, chopped
- Sea salt and black pepper to taste

Directions:
1). Preheat oven to 370°F (190°C).
2). Line muffin tray with ham slices.
3). Whisk eggs, cream, mustard, thyme, salt, and pepper.
4). Pour into ham-lined cups, 3/4 full.
5). Bake 10-15 mins, until ham is crisp and eggs cooked. Cool 5 mins. Serve.

Servings: 6

Prep time: 10 mins

Cook time: 45 mins

Nutritional value (per serving):
Calories: 150
Carbs: 1g
Protein: 12g
Saturated fat: 5g
Unsaturated fat: 3g

Sausage & Cheese Breakfast Casserole

Ingredients:

- 8 large eggs
- 1 cup heavy cream
- 1 lb ground sausage
- 1 cup shredded cheddar
- 1 cup shredded mozzarella
- 1/2 cup grated Parmesan
- 1/4 tsp garlic powder
- 1/4 tsp onion powder
- Sea salt and black pepper to taste
- 2 tbsp fresh chives, chopped

Directions:

1). Preheat oven to 350°F (175°C).

2). Cook sausage; drain fat.

3). Whisk eggs, cream, garlic, onion powder, salt, and pepper.

4). Spread sausage in a greased baking dish. Pour egg mixture.

5). Top with cheddar, mozzarella, and Parmesan.

6). Bake for 45 mins until set and golden. Cool 10 mins. Garnish with chives. Serve.

Servings: 4

Prep time: 20 mins

Cook time: 45 mins

Nutritional value (per serving):
Calories: 620
Carbs: 4g
Protein: 38g
Saturated fat: 29g
Unsaturated fat: 18g

Poached Eggs

Ingredients:
- 2 large eggs
- 1/2 tsp salt
- 3 tbsp butter

Directions:
1). Melt butter in skillet over medium heat.

2). Crack eggs into skillet, keeping yolks intact.

3). Sprinkle with salt and cook 3-4 mins until whites set, yolks runny.

4). Remove with spatula. Serve warm.

Servings: 1

Prep time: 5 mins

Cook time: 5 mins

Nutritional value (per serving):
Calories: 230

Carbs: 1g

Protein: 13g

Saturated fat: 12g

Unsaturated fat: 6g

Omelette with Cheddar Cheese

Ingredients:

- 3 large eggs
- 2 tbsp butter
- 1/2 cup shredded cheddar cheese
- Sea salt and black pepper to taste

Directions:

1). Whisk eggs in a bowl.
2). Melt butter in a skillet over medium heat.
3). Pour eggs into skillet, cook 2-3 mins until edges set.
4). Sprinkle cheese on one half, fold omelette, cook 2-3 mins until cheese melts.
5). Serve warm, seasoned with salt and pepper.

Servings: 1

Prep time: 5 mins

Cook time: 10 mins

Nutritional value (per serving):
Calories: 350
Carbs: 1g
Protein: 20g
Saturated fat: 22g
Unsaturated fat: 8g

Soft-Boiled Eggs with Sea Salt

Ingredients:
- 2 large eggs
- 1/2 tsp sea salt

Directions:
1). Boil water, gently lower eggs in.
2). Boil for 6-7 mins for runny yolk.
3). Cool eggs in ice water for 1 min, peel, and sprinkle with sea salt.

Servings: 1

Prep time: 5 mins

Cook time: 7 mins

Nutritional value (per serving):
Calories: 140
Carbs: 1g
Protein: 12g
Saturated fat: 3g
Unsaturated fat: 5g

Egg Muffins with Sausage

Ingredients:
- 8 large eggs
- 1 cup cooked sausage, crumbled
- 1/2 cup heavy cream
- 1 cup shredded cheddar cheese
- Sea salt and black pepper to taste

Directions:
1). Preheat oven to 375°F (190°C).
2). Grease muffin tray, whisk eggs, cream, salt, and pepper.
3). Divide sausage and cheese among cups, pour egg mixture.
4). Bake 20-25 mins until firm. Cool 5 mins, serve warm.

Servings: 6

Prep time: 10 mins

Cook time: 25 mins

Nutritional value (per serving):
Calories: 280
Carbs: 2g
Protein: 20g
Saturated fat: 16g
Unsaturated fat: 6g

Carnivore Pancakes (Egg and Pork Rinds)

Ingredients:

- 4 large eggs
- 1/2 cup pork rinds, crushed
- 1/4 cup heavy cream
- 1 tsp vanilla extract
- 1 tbsp butter (for cooking)

Directions:

1). Blend eggs, pork rinds, cream, and vanilla until smooth.

2). Melt butter in skillet over medium heat, pour batter.

3). Cook 2-3 mins per side until golden. Serve warm.

Servings: 2

Prep time: 5 mins

Cook time: 10 mins

Nutritional value (per serving):

Calories: 340

Carbs: 1g

Protein: 20g

Saturated fat: 16g

Unsaturated fat: 6g

Steak and Eggs

Ingredients:
- 2 ribeye steaks (8 oz each)
- 4 large eggs
- 2 tbsp butter
- Sea salt and black pepper to taste
- 1 tbsp fresh parsley, chopped (optional)

Directions:
1). Preheat skillet, melt 1 tbsp butter.
2). Season steaks, cook 4-5 mins per side. Rest steaks.
3). In same skillet, add remaining butter, fry eggs to desired doneness.
4). Serve eggs with steaks, garnish with parsley.

Servings: 2

Prep time: 10 mins

Cook time: 15 mins

Nutritional value (per serving):
Calories: 650
Carbs: 1g
Protein: 48g
Saturated fat: 25g
Unsaturated fat: 20g

Eggs Benedict with Hollandaise Sauce

Ingredients:
- 8 large eggs
- 4 slices ham
- 4 tbsp butter, divided
- Sea salt and black pepper to taste

Hollandaise sauce:
- 3 egg yolks
- 1 tbsp lemon juice
- 1/2 cup melted butter
- Sea salt to taste

Directions:
1). Whisk egg yolks and lemon juice over simmering water, slowly add melted butter until thick. Set aside.
2). Cook ham in 2 tbsp butter, set aside.
3). Poach eggs in simmering water with vinegar, 3-4 mins.
4). Assemble: place poached eggs on ham, top with hollandaise. Season with salt and pepper.

Servings: 4

Prep time: 15 mins

Cook time: 20 mins

Nutritional value (per serving):
Calories: 400
Carbs: 1g
Protein: 20g
Saturated fat: 30g
Unsaturated fat: 10g

Carnivore Breakfast Pizza (Eggs, Bacon, Cheese)

Ingredients:
- 6 large eggs
- 1 cup shredded cheese
- 6 slices bacon, cooked and crumbled
- Sea salt and black pepper to taste
- 2 tbsp butter

Directions:
1). Preheat oven to 375°F (190°C).
2). Whisk eggs, season with salt and pepper.
3). Melt butter in oven-safe skillet, pour egg mixture.
4). Cook 2-3 mins, sprinkle cheese and bacon.
5). Bake 10-15 mins until cheese is melted and eggs are set.

Servings: 4

Prep time: 10 mins

Cook time: 20 mins

Nutritional value (per serving):
Calories: 300
Carbs: 1g
Protein: 22g
Saturated fat: 18g
Unsaturated fat: 6g

Meat Lover's Breakfast Skillet
(Bacon, Sausage, Eggs)

Ingredients:
- 4 slices bacon, chopped
- 4 sausage links, sliced
- 8 large eggs
- 1 cup shredded cheese (optional)
- Sea salt and black pepper to taste
- 2 tbsp butter

Directions:
1). Cook bacon in skillet until crispy. Set aside.
2). Cook sausage in same skillet, set aside with bacon.
3). Melt butter, scramble eggs to desired doneness.
4). Mix in bacon and sausage, top with cheese if desired.

Servings: 4

Prep time: 10 mins

Cook time: 20 mins

Nutritional value (per serving):
Calories: 350
Carbs: 2g
Protein: 25g
Saturated fat: 20g
Unsaturated fat: 8g

Bone Broth Breakfast Soup

Ingredients:
- 4 cups bone broth
- 4 large eggs
- 1 cup cooked shredded chicken
- 1 tbsp butter
- Sea salt and black pepper to taste

Directions:
1). Simmer bone broth.
2). Add chicken and heat through.
3). Poach eggs in broth 3-4 mins.
4). Stir in butter, season, serve.

Servings: 4

Prep time: 10 mins

Cook time: 20 mins

Nutritional value (per serving):
Calories: 200
Carbs: 0g
Protein: 18g
Saturated fat: 6g
Unsaturated fat: 4g

Smoked Salmon and Scrambled Eggs

Ingredients:

- 4 large eggs
- 2 oz smoked salmon, chopped
- 2 tbsp heavy cream
- 1 tbsp butter
- Sea salt and black pepper to taste
- Fresh dill for garnish

Directions:

1). Whisk eggs, cream, salt, and pepper.
2). Melt butter in skillet, pour egg mixture.
3). Gently scramble eggs.
4). Add salmon before eggs fully set, stir.
5). Garnish with dill, serve.

Servings: 2

Prep time: 10 mins

Cook time: 10 mins

Nutritional value (per serving):
Calories: 200
Carbs: 1g
Protein: 15g
Saturated fat: 10g
Unsaturated fat: 5g

Cream Cheese and Egg Puffs

Ingredients:
- 6 large eggs
- 4 oz cream cheese, softened
- 1 tbsp butter, melted
- Sea salt and black pepper to taste

Directions:
1). Preheat oven to 375°F (190°C), grease muffin pan.
2). Beat eggs, mix in cream cheese, season with salt and pepper.
3). Fill muffin cups 3/4 full.
4). Drizzle melted butter over puffs.
5). Bake 20 mins until set and golden. Cool slightly before serving.

Servings: 4

Prep time: 10 mins

Cook time: 20 mins

Nutritional value (per serving):
Calories: 150
Carbs: 2g
Protein: 8g
Saturated fat: 10g
Unsaturated fat: 4g

Starters

Bacon-Wrapped Scallops

Ingredients:
- 12 large sea scallops
- 12 slices bacon
- 2 tbsp butter, melted
- Sea salt and black pepper to taste
- Lemon wedges for serving

Directions:
1). Preheat oven to 400°F (200°C).
2). Wrap each scallop in bacon, secure with toothpick.
3). Place on baking sheet, brush with butter, season.
4). Bake 15-20 mins until cooked through. Serve with lemon.

Servings: 4

Prep time: 15 mins

Cook time: 20 mins

Nutritional value (per serving):
Calories: 300
Carbs: 0g
Protein: 25g
Saturated fat: 12g
Unsaturated fat: 8g

Deviled Eggs with Bacon Bits

Ingredients:
- 6 large eggs
- 3 tbsp mayonnaise
- 1 tsp Dijon mustard
- 1/4 tsp paprika
- Sea salt and black pepper to taste
- 2 slices bacon, crumbled
- Chopped chives for garnish

Directions:
1). Boil eggs, cool, peel, and halve.
2). Mash yolks with mayonnaise, mustard, paprika, salt, and pepper.
3). Pipe yolk mixture into whites, top with bacon and chives.

Servings: 6

Prep time: 15 mins

Cook time: 10 mins

Nutritional value (per serving):
Calories: 120
Carbs: 1g
Protein: 7g
Saturated fat: 3g
Unsaturated fat: 4g

Prosciutto-Wrapped Asparagus

Ingredients:

- 1 bunch asparagus
- 12 slices prosciutto
- 1 tbsp olive oil
- Sea salt and black pepper to taste

Directions:

1). Preheat oven to 400°F (200°C).

2). Wrap asparagus in prosciutto, drizzle with oil, season.

3). Bake for 15 mins until crispy. Serve warm.

Servings: 4

Prep time: 10 mins

Cook time: 15 mins

Nutritional value (per serving):

Calories: 150

Carbs: 2g

Protein: 10g

Saturated fat: 4g

Unsaturated fat: 8g

Crispy Chicken Skins

Ingredients:
- Skins from 4 chicken breasts
- 1 tbsp olive oil
- Sea salt and black pepper to taste

Directions:
1). Preheat oven to 375°F (190°C).
2). Pat chicken skins dry, brush with oil, season.
3). Bake 45 mins until crispy. Cool slightly before serving.

Servings: 4

Prep time: 10 mins

Cook time: 45 mins

Nutritional value (per serving):
Calories: 200
Carbs: 0g
Protein: 15g
Saturated fat: 4g
Unsaturated fat: 10g

Lamb Meatballs with Mint Sauce

Ingredients:
- 1 lb ground lamb
- 1 egg
- 1/4 cup Parmesan, grated
- 2 cloves garlic, minced
- 1 tbsp mint, chopped
- 1 tbsp parsley, chopped
- Sea salt and black pepper to taste

Mint Sauce:
- 1/2 cup Greek yogurt (or lamb fat)
- 1 tbsp mint, chopped
- 1 tbsp lemon juice
- Sea salt to taste

Directions:
1). Preheat oven to 375°F (190°C).
2). Mix lamb, egg, Parmesan, garlic, mint, parsley, salt, and pepper. Shape into meatballs. Bake 20-25 mins.
3). Mix yogurt, mint, lemon juice, and salt for sauce. Serve with meatballs.

Servings: 4

Prep time: 20 mins

Cook time: 25 mins

Nutritional value (per serving):
Calories: 350
Carbs: 2g
Protein: 22g
Saturated fat: 15g
Unsaturated fat: 12g

Shrimp Cocktail (with Carnivore Sauce)

Ingredients:
- 1 lb large shrimp, peeled
- 1 lemon
- Sea salt to taste

Carnivore Sauce:
- 1/2 cup mayonnaise
- 2 tbsp horseradish
- 1 tbsp lemon juice
- 1 tsp Worcestershire sauce (optional)
- Sea salt to taste

Directions:
1). Boil water with half a lemon and salt. Cook shrimp 2-3 mins until pink.
2). Chill shrimp in ice water.
3). Mix sauce ingredients. Serve shrimp with sauce.

Servings: 4

Prep time: 10 mins

Cook time: 5 mins

Nutritional value (per serving):
Calories: 250
Carbs: 1g
Protein: 20g
Saturated fat: 5g
Unsaturated fat: 15g

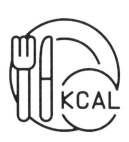

Carnivore Charcuterie Board

Ingredients:

- 8 oz prosciutto, sliced
- 8 oz salami, sliced
- 8 oz chorizo, sliced
- 8 oz smoked sausage, sliced
- 8 oz cheese (cheddar, gouda, blue cheese)
- 4 oz pâté (optional)
- 4 oz pork rinds
- 4 oz olives (optional)
- 2 oz pickles (optional)

Directions:

1). Arrange meats on a serving board.
2). Add cheese slices around the meats.
3). Place pâté in a dish (if using) and add to the board.
4). Fill spaces with pork rinds, olives, and pickles.

Servings: 6

Prep time: 15 mins

Nutritional value (per serving):
Calories: 450
Carbs: 2g
Protein: 28g
Saturated fat: 22g
Unsaturated fat: 18g

MainDishes

Ribeye Steak with Garlic Butter

Ingredients:
- 2 ribeye steaks (12 oz each)
- 2 tbsp olive oil
- Sea salt and black pepper to taste
- 4 tbsp butter
- 4 cloves garlic, minced
- 1 tbsp fresh thyme, chopped

Directions:
1). Preheat grill to high heat.
2). Rub steaks with olive oil, season with salt and pepper.
3). Grill 4-5 mins per side for medium-rare.
4). Melt butter with garlic and thyme in saucepan.
5). Let steaks rest 5 mins, drizzle with garlic butter.

Servings: 2

Prep time: 10 mins

Cook time: 15 mins

Nutritional value (per serving):
Calories: 650
Carbs: 1g
Protein: 45g
Saturated fat: 25g
Unsaturated fat: 22g

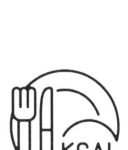

Slow Cooker Beef Brisket

Ingredients:

- 3 lb beef brisket
- 2 tbsp sea salt
- 1 tbsp black pepper
- 2 tsp smoked paprika
- 2 tsp garlic powder
- 1 tsp onion powder
- 1 cup beef broth

Directions:

1). Rub brisket with spices.
2). Place in slow cooker, pour broth around.
3). Cook on low for 8 hours.
4). Let brisket rest 10 mins, slice.

Servings: 6

Prep time: 15 mins

Cook time: 8 hours

Nutritional value (per serving):

Calories: 420
Carbs: 2g
Protein: 45g
Saturated fat: 12g
Unsaturated fat: 18g

Grilled Lamb Chops

Ingredients:

- 8 lamb chops (1 inch thick)
- 3 tbsp olive oil
- 1 tbsp rosemary, chopped
- 2 cloves garlic, minced
- Sea salt and black pepper to taste

Directions:

1). Preheat grill to medium-high.
2). Rub chops with olive oil, rosemary, garlic, salt, and pepper.
3). Grill 5-6 mins per side for medium-rare.
4). Let rest 5 mins, serve.

Servings: 4

Prep time: 10 mins

Cook time: 15 mins

Nutritional value (per serving):
Calories: 360
Carbs: 0g
Protein: 25g
Saturated fat: 12g
Unsaturated fat: 18g

Beef Tenderloin with Blue Cheese Crust

Ingredients:

- 2 lb beef tenderloin
- 2 tbsp olive oil
- Sea salt and black pepper to taste
- 4 oz blue cheese, crumbled
- 2 tbsp butter, softened
- 1 tbsp parsley, chopped

Directions:

1). Preheat oven to 400°F (200°C).
2). Rub tenderloin with olive oil, salt, and pepper.
3). Mix blue cheese, butter, and parsley.
4). Sear tenderloin, transfer to baking dish, top with cheese mixture.
5). Bake 35-40 mins, let rest 10 mins.

Servings: 4

Prep time: 15 mins

Cook time: 45 mins

Nutritional value (per serving):
Calories: 510
Carbs: 2g
Protein: 45g
Saturated fat: 22g
Unsaturated fat: 20g

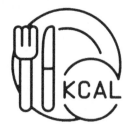

Smoked Beef Ribs

Ingredients:

- 4 beef short ribs
- 2 tbsp sea salt
- 1 tbsp black pepper
- 2 tsp garlic powder
- 1 tsp onion powder
- 1 tsp smoked paprika

Directions:

1). Preheat smoker to 225°F (107°C).

2). Rub ribs with spices.

3). Smoke for 6 hours until tender.

4). Let rest 10 mins, serve.

Servings: 4

Prep time: 15 mins

Cook time: 6 hours

Nutritional value (per serving):
Calories: 620
Carbs: 1g
Protein: 45g
Saturated fat: 20g
Unsaturated fat: 25g

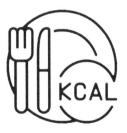

Ground Beef Carnivore Chili

Ingredients:

- 2 lbs ground beef
- 1 cup beef bone broth
- 1 tbsp smoked paprika
- 1 tbsp chili powder
- 1 tsp garlic powder
- 1 tsp onion powder
- 1 tsp sea salt
- ½ tsp black pepper

Directions:

1). Brown beef in pot. Drain fat.

2). Add broth, spices, and simmer for 45 mins to 1 hour.

3). Serve hot.

Servings: 6

Prep time: 10 mins

Cook time: 1 hour

Nutritional value (per serving):

Calories: 320

Carbs: 2g

Protein: 25g

Saturated fat: 5g

Unsaturated fat: 15g

Beef and Lamb Meatloaf

Ingredients:
- 1 lb ground beef
- 1 lb ground lamb
- 1 egg
- ½ cup Parmesan, grated
- 1 tsp garlic powder
- 1 tsp onion powder
- 1 tsp dried thyme
- 1 tsp sea salt
- ½ tsp black pepper
- 4 slices bacon, chopped

Directions:
1). Preheat oven to 350°F (175°C).
2). Mix all ingredients, shape into loaf.
3). Top with bacon, bake for 1 hour.
4). Let rest 10 mins, slice.

Servings: 6

Prep time: 15 mins

Cook time: 1 hour

Nutritional value (per serving):
Calories: 400
Carbs: 1g
Protein: 28g
Saturated fat: 16g
Unsaturated fat: 12g

Braised Short Ribs

Ingredients:

- 4 lbs beef short ribs
- 2 tbsp olive oil
- 1 cup beef bone broth
- 1 cup red wine
- 1 tbsp tomato paste
- 2 cloves garlic, minced
- 1 tsp sea salt
- ½ tsp black pepper
- 2 sprigs thyme

Directions:

1). Preheat oven to 325°F (165°C).
2). Brown ribs in Dutch oven, set aside.
3). Add garlic, broth, wine, and tomato paste, scrape browned bits.
4). Return ribs to pot, add thyme. Braise 3 hours.
5). Remove thyme, serve.

Servings: 4

Prep time: 15 mins

Cook time: 3 hours

Nutritional value (per serving):
Calories: 620
Carbs: 3g
Protein: 40g
Saturated fat: 22g
Unsaturated fat: 25g

Grilled T-Bone Steak

Ingredients:
- 2 (1 lb each) T-bone steaks
- 1 tbsp olive oil
- 1 tbsp sea salt
- 1 tsp black pepper
- 1 tsp garlic powder

Directions:
1). Preheat grill to high heat.
2). Brush steaks with olive oil, season with salt, pepper, and garlic powder.
3). Grill 6-8 mins per side for desired doneness (135°F for medium-rare).
4). Let rest 5-10 mins before serving.

Servings: 2

Prep time: 10 mins

Cook time: 15 mins

Nutritional value (per serving):
Calories: 650
Carbs: 1g
Protein: 65g
Saturated fat: 20g
Unsaturated fat: 28g

Chuck Roast with Bone Broth Gravy

Ingredients:

- 3 lbs chuck roast
- 2 tbsp olive oil
- 1 cup beef bone broth
- 1 onion, chopped
- 2 cloves garlic, minced
- 1 tbsp tomato paste
- 1 tsp sea salt
- ½ tsp black pepper
- 2 sprigs rosemary

Directions:

1). Preheat oven to 300°F (150°C).
2). Brown roast in Dutch oven, remove.
3). Sauté onion and garlic, add tomato paste.
4). Add broth and rosemary, return roast.
5). Roast 4 hours, remove rosemary, shred.

Servings: 6

Prep time: 15 mins

Cook time: 4 hours

Nutritional value (per serving):

Calories: 480
Carbs: 3g
Protein: 45g
Saturated fat: 15g
Unsaturated fat: 20g

Garlic Herb Prime Rib

Ingredients:

- 4 lb prime rib roast
- 3 tbsp sea salt
- 2 tbsp black pepper
- 2 tbsp garlic, minced
- 1 tbsp rosemary
- 1 tbsp thyme
- 4 tbsp butter, melted

Directions:

1). Preheat oven to 450°F (230°C).
2). Rub roast with seasoning, place fat-side up.
3). Roast 15 mins, reduce to 325°F, cook 1 hour 45 mins (135°F for medium-rare).
4). Baste with butter halfway through, let rest 15 mins.

Servings: 6

Prep time: 20 mins

Cook time: 2 hours

Nutritional value (per serving):

Calories: 700
Carbs: 2g
Protein: 60g
Saturated fat: 25g
Unsaturated fat: 35g

Veal Cutlets with Lemon Butter Sauce

Ingredients:

- 4 veal cutlets
- 2 tbsp butter
- 1 lemon, juiced and zested
- 1 tbsp capers, drained
- 1 tbsp parsley, chopped
- Sea salt and black pepper to taste

Directions:

1). Season cutlets with salt and pepper.

2). Sear cutlets in butter, remove.

3). Add lemon juice, zest, and capers to skillet. Spoon sauce over cutlets.

4). Cook 1-2 mins, garnish with parsley.

Servings: 4

Prep time: 10 mins

Cook time: 20 mins

Nutritional value (per serving):
Calories: 300
Carbs: 2g
Protein: 36g
Saturated fat: 6g
Unsaturated fat: 10g

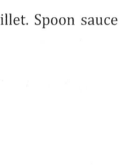

Lamb Shoulder Roast

Ingredients:

- 3-4 lb lamb shoulder roast
- 3 cloves garlic, minced
- 2 tbsp olive oil
- 2 tsp rosemary, chopped
- 2 tsp thyme, chopped
- Sea salt and black pepper to taste

Directions:

1). Preheat oven to 325°F (165°C).

2). Rub roast with garlic, oil, and herbs.

3). Roast 2 hours, uncover and roast 30 mins more.

4). Let rest 10-15 mins before slicing.

Servings: 6

Prep time: 15 mins

Cook time: 2 hours 30 mins

Nutritional value (per serving):
Calories: 450
Carbs: 1g
Protein: 42g
Saturated fat: 16g
Unsaturated fat: 20g

Roast Chicken with Herb Butter

Ingredients:

- 1 whole chicken (4 lbs)
- ½ cup butter, softened
- 2 tbsp rosemary, chopped
- 2 tbsp thyme, chopped
- 4 cloves garlic, minced
- Sea salt and black pepper to taste
- 1 lemon, halved

Directions:

1). Preheat oven to 375°F (190°C).

2). Rub chicken with herb butter, place lemon halves in cavity.

3). Roast 1 hour 30 mins, let rest 10 mins before carving.

Servings: 6

Prep time: 15 mins

Cook time: 1 hour 30 mins

Nutritional value (per serving):
Calories: 450
Carbs: 1g
Protein: 35g
Saturated fat: 14g
Unsaturated fat: 18g

Duck Breast with Crispy Skin

Ingredients:

- 4 duck breasts, skin on
- Sea salt and black pepper to taste
- 1 tsp garlic powder
- 1 tsp dried thyme

Directions:

1). Score duck breast skin, season with salt, pepper, garlic powder, and thyme.
2). Cook skin-side down in cold skillet, medium heat, until crispy (8-10 mins).
3). Flip, roast in oven at 400°F (200°C) for 6-10 mins.
4). Let rest 5 mins, slice.

Servings: 4

Prep time: 10 mins

Cook time: 25 mins

Nutritional value (per serving):
Calories: 360
Carbs: 0g
Protein: 30g
Saturated fat: 5g
Unsaturated fat: 16g

Chicken Thighs in Cream Sauce

Ingredients:
- 8 chicken thighs, skin on
- Sea salt and black pepper to taste
- 2 tbsp butter
- 1 cup heavy cream
- ½ cup chicken broth
- 1 tbsp Dijon mustard
- 4 cloves garlic, minced
- 2 tbsp parsley, chopped

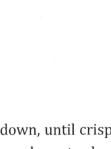

Directions:
1). Sear chicken thighs in butter, skin-side down, until crispy.
2). Remove, sauté garlic, add cream, broth, and mustard.
3). Return chicken to skillet, bake at 375°F (190°C) for 30 mins. Garnish with parsley.

Servings: 4

Prep time: 10 mins

Cook time: 45 mins

Nutritional value (per serving):
Calories: 520
Carbs: 2g
Protein: 36g
Saturated fat: 24g
Unsaturated fat: 12g

Bacon-Wrapped Chicken Breasts

Ingredients:

- 4 chicken breasts
- 8 slices bacon
- Sea salt and black pepper to taste
- 1 tsp garlic powder
- 1 tsp paprika

Directions:

1). Season chicken breasts with salt, pepper, garlic powder, and paprika.
2). Wrap each breast in bacon, secure with toothpicks.
3). Bake at 375°F (190°C) for 25-30 mins.

Servings: 4

Prep time: 10 mins

Cook time: 30 mins

Nutritional value (per serving):

Calories: 360
Carbs: 1g
Protein: 40g
Saturated fat: 10g
Unsaturated fat: 14g

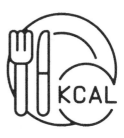

Turkey Drumsticks with Garlic Butter

Ingredients:
- 4 turkey drumsticks
- Sea salt and black pepper to taste
- 4 tbsp butter, melted
- 4 cloves garlic, minced
- 1 tbsp rosemary, chopped
- 1 tbsp thyme, chopped

Directions:
1). Rub drumsticks with salt and pepper, brush with garlic butter.
2). Roast at 350°F (175°C) for 1 hour 30 mins, basting every 30 mins.

Servings: 4

Prep time: 10 mins

Cook time: 1 hour 30 mins

Nutritional value (per serving):
Calories: 480
Carbs: 1g
Protein: 45g
Saturated fat: 12g
Unsaturated fat: 18g

Grilled Chicken Wings

Ingredients:

- 2 lbs chicken wings
- 2 tbsp olive oil
- 1 tbsp garlic powder
- 1 tsp sea salt
- 1 tsp black pepper
- 1 tsp paprika
- 1 tsp dried thyme

Directions:

1). Toss wings in olive oil and spices.
2). Grill 20-25 mins until crispy, turning occasionally.

Servings: 4

Prep time: 10 mins

Cook time: 25 mins

Nutritional value (per serving):
Calories: 380
Carbs: 0g
Protein: 30g
Saturated fat: 6g
Unsaturated fat: 22g

Chicken Alfredo (Carnivore Style)

Ingredients:

- 4 chicken breasts
- 2 tbsp butter
- 1 cup heavy cream
- 1 cup Parmesan, grated
- 2 cloves garlic, minced
- 1 tsp sea salt
- 1 tsp black pepper

Directions:

1). Cook chicken breasts, remove.
2). Sauté garlic, add cream and Parmesan.
3). Return chicken, cook 2-3 mins in sauce.

Servings: 4

Prep time: 15 mins

Cook time: 25 mins

Nutritional value (per serving):

Calories: 600
Carbs: 3g
Protein: 45g
Saturated fat: 28g
Unsaturated fat: 14g

Lemon Garlic Chicken Skewers

Ingredients:

- 1 lb chicken breasts, cubed
- 2 lemons, juiced and zested
- 3 cloves garlic, minced
- 2 tbsp olive oil
- Sea salt and black pepper to taste
- 2 tbsp parsley, chopped

Directions:

1). Marinate chicken in lemon, garlic, and olive oil for 30 mins.

2). Grill 10-15 mins on skewers.

Servings: 4

Prep time: 15 mins

Cook time: 20 mins

Nutritional value (per serving):

Calories: 210

Carbs: 2g

Protein: 28g

Saturated fat: 2g

Unsaturated fat: 8g

Stuffed Turkey Thighs

Ingredients:
- 4 turkey thighs
- 1 lb ground pork
- ½ cup Parmesan, grated
- ¼ cup parsley, chopped
- 2 cloves garlic, minced
- Sea salt and black pepper to taste
- 2 tbsp olive oil

Directions:
Stuff thighs with pork mixture, sear, then roast at 375°F (190°C) for 1 hour 20 mins.

Servings: 4

Prep time: 20 mins

Cook time: 1 hour 30 mins

Nutritional value (per serving):
Calories: 450
Carbs: 2g
Protein: 50g
Saturated fat: 10g
Unsaturated fat: 12g

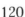

BBQ Chicken Drumsticks

Ingredients:

- 8 chicken drumsticks
- 2 tbsp olive oil
- 1 tsp sea salt
- 1 tsp black pepper
- 1 tbsp smoked paprika
- 1 tsp garlic powder
- 1 tsp onion powder
- 1 cup sugar-free BBQ sauce

Directions:

Bake drumsticks at 400°F (200°C) for 40 mins, then brush with BBQ sauce and bake 10 mins more.

Servings: 4

Prep time: 10 mins

Cook time: 50 mins

Nutritional value (per serving):

Calories: 310

Carbs: 4g

Protein: 28g

Saturated fat: 4g

Unsaturated fat: 8g

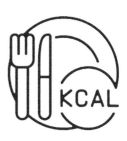

Garlic Shrimp Scampi

Ingredients:

- 1 lb shrimp
- 4 tbsp butter
- 4 cloves garlic, minced
- ¼ cup chicken broth
- ¼ cup lemon juice
- Sea salt and black pepper to taste
- Parsley, chopped

Directions:

Sauté shrimp in garlic butter, add broth and lemon juice.

Servings: 4

Prep time: 10 mins

Cook time: 10 mins

Nutritional value (per serving):

Calories: 210
Carbs: 2g
Protein: 24g
Saturated fat: 9g
Unsaturated fat: 7g

Salmon Fillet with Dill Sauce

Ingredients:

- 4 salmon fillets (6 oz each)
- Sea salt and black pepper
- 2 tbsp olive oil
- ¼ cup sour cream
- 1 tbsp dill, chopped
- 1 tbsp lemon juice

Directions:
1). Season salmon, sear skin-side down in oil 3-4 mins.

2). Bake at 400°F for 8-10 mins.

3). Mix sour cream, lemon juice, and dill. Serve with salmon.

Servings: 4

Prep time: 10 mins

Cook time: 15 mins

Nutritional value (per serving):
Calories: 310
Carbs: 2g
Protein: 25g
Saturated fat: 6g
Unsaturated fat: 12g

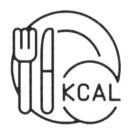

Crab Cakes (Carnivore Style)

Ingredients:

- 1 lb crab meat
- 2 large eggs, beaten
- ¼ cup crushed pork rinds
- 2 tbsp mayo
- 1 tbsp Dijon mustard
- 1 tbsp lemon juice
- 1 tsp Old Bay seasoning
- 2 tbsp butter

Directions:

1). Mix crab, eggs, pork rinds, mayo, mustard, lemon juice, and seasoning.

2). Shape into 8 patties.

3). Cook in butter 4-5 mins per side.

Servings: 4

Prep time: 15 mins

Cook time: 20 mins

Nutritional value (per serving):
Calories: 220
Carbs: 1g
Protein: 20g
Saturated fat: 8g
Unsaturated fat: 5g

Grilled Ribeye Steak with Rosemary Butter

Ingredients:

- 4 ribeye steaks (8 oz each)
- 2 tbsp olive oil
- 4 cloves garlic, minced
- 2 tsp rosemary, chopped
- 4 tbsp butter, softened
- 1 tsp lemon juice

Directions:

1). Rub steaks with olive oil, garlic, rosemary, salt, and pepper.

2). Grill 4-5 mins per side.

3). Top with rosemary butter.

Servings: 4

Prep time: 10 mins

Cook time: 15 mins

Nutritional value (per serving):
Calories: 450
Carbs: 1g
Protein: 38g
Saturated fat: 18g
Unsaturated fat: 14g

Blackened Catfish

Ingredients:
- 4 catfish fillets
- 2 tbsp olive oil
- 1 tbsp smoked paprika
- 1 tsp garlic powder
- 1 tsp onion powder
- 1 tsp oregano
- 1 tsp thyme
- ½ tsp cayenne pepper

Directions:
1). Rub fillets with oil and spices.
2). Bake at 400°F for 12-15 mins.

Servings: 4

Prep time: 10 mins

Cook time: 15 mins

Nutritional value (per serving):
Calories: 250
Carbs: 2g
Protein: 35g
Saturated fat: 2g
Unsaturated fat: 10g

Shrimp and Crab Boil

Ingredients:
- 1 lb shrimp
- 1 lb crab legs
- 4 cups water
- 1 lemon, halved
- 4 cloves garlic, smashed
- 2 tbsp Old Bay seasoning
- 1 tbsp sea salt
- 4 tbsp butter, melted

Directions:
1). Boil water with lemon, garlic, Old Bay seasoning, and salt.
2). Cook crab legs for 10 minutes.
3). Add shrimp and cook for an additional 5 minutes.
4). Drain and serve with melted butter.

Servings: 6

Prep time: 20 mins

Cook time: 30 mins

Nutritional value (per serving):
Calories: 350
Carbs: 3g
Protein: 38g
Saturated fat: 10g
Unsaturated fat: 12g

Grilled Chicken Skewers

Ingredients:

- 1.5 lbs chicken breast, cubed
- ¼ cup olive oil
- 2 tbsp lemon juice
- 1 tbsp dried oregano
- 1 tsp garlic powder

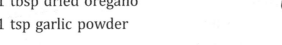

Directions:

1). Marinate chicken in oil, lemon, oregano, garlic.

2). Grill on skewers for 10 minutes.

Servings: 4

Prep time: 20 mins

Cook time: 10 mins

Nutritional value (per serving):

Calories: 250

Carbs: 1g

Protein: 35g

Saturated fat: 3g

Unsaturated fat: 7g

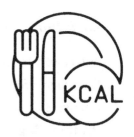

Herb Butter Roasted Chicken Wings

Ingredients:

- 2 lbs chicken wings
- ¼ cup butter, melted
- 2 tbsp fresh rosemary, chopped
- 2 tbsp fresh thyme, chopped
- 1 tsp garlic powder

Directions:

1). Toss wings in butter, herbs, and garlic powder.

2). Roast at 400°F for 40-45 minutes, turning halfway.

Servings: 4

Prep time: 10 mins

Cook time: 45 mins

Nutritional value (per serving):

Calories: 320

Carbs: 0g

Protein: 25g

Saturated fat: 10g

Unsaturated fat: 12g

Additional Resources

Expanding your knowledge about the carnivore diet can empower you to make informed decisions and deepen your understanding of its principles and effects. Below is a list of recommended literature and studies that offer valuable insights into the science and practical application of the carnivore diet.

Recommended Literature

1. "The Carnivore Diet" by Dr. Shawn Baker

In this book, Dr. Baker shares his extensive experience with the carnivore diet, including scientific explanations, personal anecdotes, and practical advice for adopting this way of eating. He addresses common concerns and provides guidance on how to optimize health through a meat-based diet.

2. "The Carnivore Code" by Dr. Paul Saladino

Dr. Saladino delves into the evolutionary and scientific rationale behind the carnivore diet. He explores how eliminating plant foods can improve health and discusses the potential benefits for autoimmune conditions, mental health, and chronic diseases.

3. "Nutrition and Physical Degeneration" by Dr. Weston A. Price

Although not exclusively about the carnivore diet, this classic work examines the dietary habits of various indigenous populations consuming traditional diets rich in animal foods. Dr. Price's observations highlight the connection between diet and health across different cultures.

4. "Fiber Menace" by Konstantin Monastyrsky

This book challenges conventional wisdom about fiber and its role in digestive health. Monastyrsky presents an alternative perspective that aligns with some of the principles of the carnivore diet regarding fiber intake.

5. "Deep Nutrition: Why Your Genes Need Traditional Food" by Dr. Catherine Shanahan

Dr. Shanahan discusses the importance of traditional diets, including the consumption of animal products, for optimal genetic expression and overall health. The book provides insights into how modern dietary changes have impacted human health.

Key Scientific Studies

1. Smith, M.D., & Wald, J. (2021). "Nutritional Adequacy of a Carnivore Diet in Adults." Journal of Nutrition and Metabolism, 2021, Article ID 8836852.

This study evaluates the nutritional content of a carnivore diet and its effects on adult health markers, concluding that with careful planning, the diet can meet most essential nutrient requirements.

2. Mancini, J.G., et al. (2016). "Effects of a High-Protein Ketogenic Diet on Hunger, Appetite, and Weight Loss in Obese Men Feeding Ad Libitum." American Journal of Clinical Nutrition, 103(2), 489–498.

Investigates how high-protein, low-carb diets affect hunger and weight loss, providing insights relevant to the carnivore diet's impact on satiety and calorie intake.

3. Bollinger, T.W., & Hsu, Y. (2019). "Low-Carbohydrate Diets and Cardiovascular Risk Factors: A Meta-Analysis of Randomized Controlled Trials." Nutrients, 11(11), 2580.

Analyzes multiple studies to assess how low-carb diets influence cardiovascular health, which can help understand potential effects of the carnivore diet.

4. Zang, Y., et al. (2015). "Gut Microbiota Composition Associated with Clostridium difficile Infection and Treatment." Scientific Reports, 5, 15088.

While not directly about the carnivore diet, this study sheds light on how diet influences gut microbiota, a relevant topic for understanding changes that may occur when adopting an all-meat diet.

5. Heilbronn, L.K., et al. (2005). "Glucose Tolerance and Skeletal Muscle Gene Expression in Response to Alternate-Day Fasting." Obesity Research, 13(3), 574–581.

Explores metabolic responses to dietary changes, providing context for how the carnivore diet might affect glucose metabolism and insulin sensitivity.

Online Resources and Communities

Revero (formerly MeatRx)

A platform founded by Dr. Shawn Baker offering resources, success stories, and community support for those interested in the carnivore diet.

The Carnivore Diet Reddit Community

An active online forum where individuals share experiences, ask questions, and provide support related to the carnivore lifestyle.

Podcast Episodes

"The Joe Rogan Experience" featuring Dr. Shawn Baker and Dr. Paul Saladino

These episodes delve into the details of the carnivore diet, with discussions on health benefits, scientific evidence, and personal experiences.

YouTube Channels

"Primal Edge Health"

Provides videos on carnivore diet topics, recipes, and interviews with experts in the field.

"Carnivore MD"

Hosted by Dr. Paul Saladino, offering insights into the science behind the diet and addressing common questions.

Research Databases

PubMed

An extensive database of biomedical literature where you can search for the latest research studies on the carnivore diet, ketogenic diets, and related topics.

Google Scholar

A comprehensive resource for accessing academic papers, theses, and scholarly articles to further explore scientific findings related to the diet.

Made in the USA
Monee, IL
06 January 2025

76172202R00075